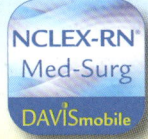
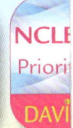

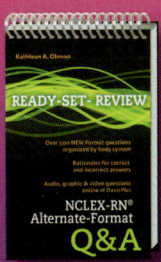
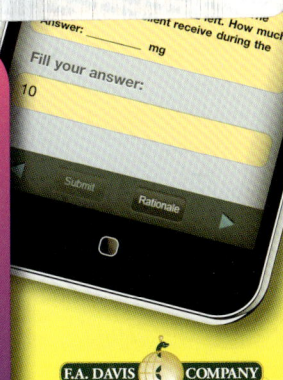

Contacts • Phone/E-Mail

Name	
Ph:	e-mail:
Name	
Ph:	e-mail:
Name	
Ph:	e-mail:
Name	
Ph:	e-mail:
Name	
Ph:	e-mail:
Name	
Ph:	e-mail:
Name	
Ph:	e-mail:
Name	
Ph:	e-mail:
Name	
Ph:	e-mail:
Name	
Ph:	e-mail:
Name	
Ph:	e-mail:
Name	
Ph:	e-mail:

NCLEX-RN Overview

■ The National Council Licensure Examination for Registered Nurses (NCLEX-RN) measures the knowledge and abilities necessary for entry-level nurses.

- It is administered by computer-adaptive testing (CAT), which individualizes tests to match the unique competencies of each test taker.
- Each exam adheres to the NCLEX-RN Test Plan, which describes the content and scope of RN competencies.
- Practices basic to nursing (nursing process, caring, teaching, learning, communication, documentation) are integrated throughout, and most questions require application and analysis of information.

NCLEX-RN Test Plan: Distribution of Content

Patient Needs and Percentage of Items

Safe and Effective Care Environment	
• Management of Care	16%–22%
• Safety/Infection Control	8%–14%
Health Promotion and Maintenance	6%–12%
Psychosocial Integrity	6%–12%
Physiological Integrity	
• Basic Care/Comfort	6%–12%
• Pharmacological/Parenteral Therapies	13%–19%
• Reduction of Risk Potential	10%–16%
• Physiological Adaptation	11%–17%

Taking the NCLEX-RN Test on a Computer

- You will receive general information about the exam and the testing center. Your time spent on this will not count.
- You will take a tutorial on how to use the computer to answer the questions on the NCLEX-RN. Your answers will not count toward your score, but the time you take will be subtracted from the total 6 hr you have for the exam.
- You will then be presented with real NCLEX-RN items; there will be between 75 and 265 items. The test ends when it is 95% certain your ability is ↑ or ↓ the passing standard.
- Answers may be selected or deleted several times if desired before confirming a final answer. You must answer every question. You cannot return to a previous question.
- A time-remaining clock is in the screen's upper right-hand corner.
- A calculator on the computer is available for calculations.

Go to www.NCSBN.org to access an NCLEX tutorial to practice multiple-choice and alternate format items on the computer.

Critical Thinking

Definition, Influences, and Uses

- **Definition of critical thinking:** Cognitive technique in which you reflect on and analyze your thoughts, actions, and decisions.
- **Intellectual standards that influence critical thinking:** Focused, methodical, clear, deliberate, logical, relevant, accurate, and precise.
- **Processes that require critical thinking:** Test taking, nursing process, problem solving, decision making, diagnostic reasoning.

Maximize Your Critical-Thinking Abilities

Action	Benefit
Be positive: Be optimistic.	
• **Maintain a positive mental attitude:** Replace negative thoughts with positive ones.	↑ Positive thinking and ↓ negative thinking that can interfere with learning.
Be calm: Control anxious feelings.	
• **Use relaxation techniques:** Practice breathing exercises and guided imagery.	↓ Anxiety. ↑ Control in relation to intellectual tasks.
Be inquisitive: Question and investigate.	
• **Ask the questions: How? Why? What?** (e.g., "How does Colace promote a bowel movement?" "Why does BP drop with hemorrhage?")	↑ Ability to determine significance of information. ↑ Understanding and retention of information. ↑ Ability to apply information.

Continued

Action	Benefit
Be persistent: Follow a course of action.	
• **Develop self-discipline:** Be logical and organized. • **Develop perseverance:** Adhere to a preset study schedule; remain determined. • **Maintain motivation:** Set short- and long-term goals; divide tasks into steps; reward yourself.	↑ Control over variables associated with thinking. ↓ Procrastination, increases enthusiasm. ↑ Efficiency of time management. ↓ Stress of making purposeful daily study decisions, inspires action. ↑ Goal-directed behavior.
Be creative: Be innovative and resourceful.	
• **Develop open-mindedness:** Compartmentalize identified beliefs, opinions, biases, stereotypes, prejudices. • **Develop comfort with ambiguity:** Recognize there is more than one way to perform a task or achieve a goal. • **Develop independent thought:** Consider all possibilities and arrive at an autonomous conclusion. • **Take risks:** Implement unique interventions within the definition of nursing practice and safety guidelines.	↑ Openness to different perspectives; ↓ egocentric thinking; ↑ nonjudgmental thinking or practice. ↑ Comprehension, synthesis, Interpretation, analysis of information; promotes practice based on principles; ↑ innovation. ↑ Ability to synthesize, summarize, conceptualize; promotes practice based on principles.
Be reflective: Explore and assess thoughtfully.	
• **Develop courage:** Confront difficult tasks (e.g., reviewing mistakes) with a nonjudgmental attitude. • **Develop humility:** Admit your limitations—defensive thinking promotes negativity, which closes the mind. • **Use retrospective reviews:** Recall information or event to rediscover or explore its meaning; conduct internally or with others.	• Removes negative emotions from the task; ↑ positive thinking. • Allows an open mind to explore and acquire information; permits nonjudgmental review of mistakes. • Identifies strengths, weaknesses, and gaps in knowledge; ↑ understanding of relationships between information and its application; ↓ future mistakes.

General Study Skills

- Set goals.
- Take class notes.
- Manage your time.
- Control internal and external distractions.
- Establish a routine.
- Simulate a school environment.
- Prepare for class.
- Balance sacrifices and rewards.

Use Techniques Appropriate for Learning Domains

Action	Benefit
Cognitive domain (thinking): Knowing, comprehending, applying, analyzing, synthesizing, evaluating.	
• Use all your senses. • Use memorization techniques. • Put information into own words. • Apply information in new situations.	↑ Reception of information. ↑ Retention of basic information. ↑ Understanding. Encourages correct use of information.
Affective domain (feeling): Receiving, valuing, organizing, characterizing.	
• Observe role models. • Explore feelings, beliefs, and values. • Integrate values into philosophy of life.	↑ Sensitivity. ↑ Self-disclosure and growth. ↑ Consistency in actions; allows for self-actualization.
Psychomotor domain (doing): Imitating, manipulating, developing precision, articulating, naturalizing.	
• Observe others performing a skill. • Manipulate equipment while doing procedures. • Include speed and timing when practicing skills. • Practice skills repeatedly.	Identifies steps of a skill. Transfers information from head to hands. Promotes proficiency through repetition. Perfects the skill; naturalization occurs when skill becomes automatic.

How to Remember and Recall Information: Commit Facts to Memory

Action	Benefit	Example
Memorization: Repeatedly reciting out loud, reviewing in your mind, writing it down.	Repetition ↓ retention of information.	Lists on index cards: Steps of a procedure; signs of a specific electrolyte imbalance. Flash cards: Drug classification on one side and action on reverse side; medical terminology on one side and definition on reverse side.
Alphabet cues: Combination of significant letters.	Each letter prompts recall of specific information.	The three Ps—Cardinal signs of diabetes mellitus: • **Polyuria:** Increased secretion/excretion of urine. • **Polydipsia:** Excessive thirst. • **Polyphagia:** Eating excessive amounts of food.
Acronyms: Word formed from the first letters of a series of facts.	Each letter jolts retrieval of specific information.	RACE: Procedure for a fire in a health-care facility: • **R**escue people in immediate danger. • **A**ctivate the fire alarm. • **C**onfine the fire. • **E**vacuate people to a safe area.
Mnemonics: A phrase, motto, verse.	Technique prompts recall of specific information.	"There are 15 grains of sugar in 1 graham (gram) cracker." This sentence should help you remember that 15 grains are equivalent to 1 gram.

Action	Benefit	Example
Explore how or why information is relevant and valuable.	Significant information is more likely remembered.	Elevation of an extremity reduces peripheral edema. • How: Hand held above elbow and shoulder ↑ venous return via gravity, which ↓ edema.
Study in small groups.	Sharing and listening ↑ understanding and corrects misinformation.	Discussing differences between hyper- and hypoglycemia. • Debating the pros and cons of breastfeeding. • Identify more correct things the nurse should do, in addition to the correct answer presented in a test question.

How to Manipulate Information: Apply, Solve, Modify, and Use Information

Action	Benefit	Example
Relate new information to prior learning.	Placing information within a personal frame of reference makes information more meaningful.	Pathophysiology of diabetes should build on normal physiology of the pancreas. • Placing patient in left side-lying position after liver biopsy should build on the fact that pressure compresses blood vessels, which supports homeostasis, preventing hemorrhage.
Recognize commonalities.	Application of information to similar situations ↑ learning.	Actions that use the principle of gravity: • Enema instillation, elevation of extremity to limit edema, high Fowler position to promote respirations.

How to Analyze Information: Examine the Organization, Structure, and Interrelationships of Information

Action	Benefit	Example
Recognize differences.	↑ Ability to analyze and discriminate significance of information.	• Variety of causes that can ↑ BP: Hypervolemia, rigid arterial walls, emotional stress.
Practice test taking.	Reinforces learning; builds endurance; ↑ test-taking and time-management skills; ↑ testing comfort	• Answer questions at the end of a chapter. • Take a simulated test in an NCLEX prep book. • Take a simulated NCLEX test on a computer.
Review rationales for all options.	Reinforces concepts and principles; ↑ new learning; strengthens critical thinking; corrects misinformation.	• Review why the correct answer is correct. • Review why the incorrect options are incorrect. • Look up additional information in textbooks.
Modify test questions.	Identifying commonalities and differences provides more opportunities for exploring content.	• Change a key word in a stem to change the focus: "Identify patient adaptation associated with acute pain." • Change the word *acute* to *chronic* and then identify if any options apply.
Analyze your performance.	Analysis identifies areas of strength, gaps in knowledge, information-processing errors, effectiveness of educated guesses, plans for future study.	• Use the self-evaluation tools presented in Tab 8, TOOLS to identify performance trends, information-processing errors, and knowledge deficits. • Use the Corrective Action Plan presented in Tab 8, TOOLS to design an individualized plan to meet your educational needs to maximize future test success.

Test-Taking and Study Tips

See enclosed disk for 160 examples of questions demonstrating the 15 test-taking tips and alternate format questions.

Identify Positive Polarity in a Stem
Correct answer is in accord with a truth, fact, principle, or action that should be done; it attempts to determine if you can understand, apply, or differentiate correct information.

- **Study Tip:** Review content being tested; identify additional things the nurse should do.

Identify Negative Polarity in a Stem
Correct answer reflects something that is false; the words *except*, *not*, *contraindicated*, *unacceptable*, *least*, *avoid*, *violate*, *untrue*, *side effect*, and *exception* indicate negative polarity. If three answers appear correct, you may have missed the negative word in the stem.
- **Study Tip:** Change a negative word to a positive word, and then answer the question.

Identify Words That Set a Priority
Correct answer is what should be done first; the words *initial*, *main*, *primary*, *initially*, *greatest*, *best*, *first*, *most*, and *priority* require ranking of options from most to least desirable. If unable to identify correct answer, eliminate least desirable option and repeat again until left with a final option.

- **Study Tip:** After selecting correct answer, select what action should be done next.

Identify Opposites in Options
When two options reflect extremes on a continuum, frequently one of them is the correct answer; opposites may be obvious or obscure.

- **Study Tip:** Examples of opposites: *hypo-* vs. *hyper-*; *increase* vs. *decrease*; *brady-* vs. *tachy-*; identify what is associated with the incorrect opposite—for example, tachycardia is associated with hyperthyroidism vs. bradycardia is associated with hypothyroidism.

Identify Key Words in a Stem
Identify important word or phrase that modifies another word such as early vs. late signs of shock.
- **Study Tip:** Change key words in stem; this changes the focus of the question and provides more opportunities for learning.

Identify Patient-Centered Options

Correct answers testing principles in the affective domain focus on feelings, choices, empowerment, and preferences.

■ **Study Tip:** Examples of patient-centered options: Acknowledging: "Losing your independence must be difficult." Offering a choice: "Would you like your bath at 7 or 10 today?" Empowering: Encourage patient to write down questions for the primary health-care provider. Determining preferences: "What foods do you like to eat?"

Identify Equally Plausible Options

When two options are similar and one is not better than the other, generally both are incorrect.

■ **Study Tip:** Identify other equally plausible facts related to either the three incorrect options or the correct answer.

Identify Options With "Absolute" Terms

The words *all, just, none, only, never, every,* and *always* have no exceptions; one of these before a statement that is true generally makes it an incorrect option. Options with absolute terms (also called *specific determiners*) are more often incorrect.

■ **Study Tip:** Examples of options to be eliminated: "Always position an infant prone" and "Just prescription drugs can cause interactions"; exceptions include always maintaining an airway and focusing on the patient.

Identify the Global Option

A global option is a broad, general statement, whereas the three other options are specific and inherently are included under the mantle of the global option.

■ **Study Tip:** What else can be included under the global option?

Identify Options That Deny Patient's Feelings, Needs, Concerns

Options that deny feelings, give false reassurance, focus on nurse, encourage cheerfulness, or change the subject cut off communication and should be eliminated.

■ **Study Tip:** Examples of options to be eliminated: Denies feelings: "Don't cry. It's not so bad." False reassurance: "You'll feel better tomorrow." Focuses on the nurse: "The thought of dying would frighten me." Cheerfulness: "Cheer up. You are getting better."

Identify the Unique Option

When three options are similar in some way and one is different, the unique option often is the correct answer; for example, three options promote a bowel movement while the correct answer causes diarrhea.

- **Study Tip:** Identify additional similar or different examples of correct and incorrect options.

Identify Clues in a Stem

A word(s) in the stem that is identical, similar, paraphrased, or closely related to a word(s) in an option is called a *clang*; a clang can be obvious or obscure. Generally, an option with a clang is the correct answer.

- **Study Tip:** Identify a similar word(s) that relates to an important word in the stem such as the word *movement* in a stem—consider similar words such as *activity* and *mobility* that may be found in an option.

Identify Duplicate Facts in Options

If two or more facts are in each option and identical or similar facts are in at least two of the four options, and you can identify at least one fact that is correct or incorrect, you can eliminate at least two options.

- **Study Tip:** Identify additional facts that may be correct.

Use Maslow to Identify Correct Option

Answer the question in light of Maslow's hierarchy of needs; basic physiological needs are first-level needs that are a priority and are followed by needs associated with safety and security (second), love and belonging (third), self-esteem (fourth), and self-actualization (fifth).

- **Study Tip:** Identify an intervention associated with each level of Maslow's hierarchy of needs in relation to the question.

Use Multiple Test-Taking Tips

- First analyze the stem for one or more test-taking tips. Then analyze the options for one or more test-taking tips. When you focus on what the stem is asking and eliminate options from consideration, you maximize the ability to select the correct answer.
- **Study Tip:** Practice answering questions at the end of a chapter or in test-taking books using the presented test-taking tips.

Alternate Format Questions and Test-Taking Tips

- These questions evaluate certain knowledge more effectively than the typical multiple-choice question.
- They supplement multiple-choice questions, which remain the majority of questions. Any format, including the standard multiple-choice question, may include a chart, table, or graphic image.
- They are scored as either right or wrong, and partial credit is not given.

Ordered Response (Drag-and-Drop) Question

■ Presents a scenario or makes a statement, and then lists a variety of actions or factors (usually five) that must be placed in sequence.

■ The sequence chosen must be identical to the correct sequence to receive credit.

■ **Test-Taking Tip:**
1. Identify the action or factor you believe should be first.
2. Identify the action or factor you believe should be last.
3. Evaluate the remaining actions or factors and determine which one goes second and which one should be next to last.
4. The remaining action or factor is placed third.

Fill-in-the-Blank (Calculation) Question

■ Requires manipulation, interpretations, or solving a problem based on presented information.

■ Requires an intellectual skill such as computing a drug dosage, calculating an input and output (I&O), or determining the amount of IV solution to be given.

■ The recorded answer must be identical to the correct answer to receive credit.

■ You do not have to type in the unit of measurement.

■ **Test-Taking Tip:**
1. Recall information related to the question such as memorized equivalents or formulas before attempting to answer the question; this taps your knowledge first.
2. Then attempt to perform the mathematical calculation to answer the question.

Multiple-Response Question

■ Asks a question and then lists several responses.

■ You must identify the correct responses. All correct responses (usually two or more) must be selected to receive credit.

■ **Test-Taking Tip:**
1. Before looking at presented options, quickly review information you know about the topic. This taps your knowledge first and limits confusion after looking at presented options.
2. Compare your list with presented options. Some of your recalled information should match.
3. Review the remaining presented options and determine if they are applicable. If you look at the presented options first, eliminate at least one or two you believe are wrong.
4. Identify at least one or two you believe are correct.
5. Evaluate the remaining options, and determine if they are correct or not.

Hot-Spot Question

■ Asks a question in relation to a graphic image, picture, chart, or table.
■ You must identify a location on the illustration that answers the question.
■ Your answer must mirror the correct answer exactly to receive credit.
  ■ **Test-Taking Tip:**
    1. Read the question carefully to identify exactly what the question is asking. This limits misinterpretation and confusion.
    2. When questions reflect anatomy and physiology, close your eyes, visualize the area, briefly recall the significant structures and functions, and then look at the picture.
    3. When questions involve graphs or tables, first break them into segments for analysis and then review them as a whole.

Exhibit Question

■ Presents a problem and then provides an exhibit that has several tabs. It often resembles sections in a patient's clinical record.
■ Each tab has to be clicked to retrieve information contained within the tab.
■ The data must be analyzed and the significant information gleaned from the material presented to eliminate incorrect options and then select the correct option.
■ These questions require the highest level of critical thinking (analysis and synthesis).
  ■ **Test-Taking Tip:**
    1. Identify what the question is asking, then click each tab to collect data.
    2. Dissect, analyze, and compare and contrast the information collected in light of what the question is asking. Extensive information must be recalled from your body of knowledge and compared to the information in context of the situation presented in the question.

Common Human Responses and Related Nursing Care
    Vital Signs
    Fever
    Constipation
    Diarrhea
    Hemorrhage
    Shock
    Infection
    Inflammatory Response
    Nausea and Vomiting
    Deficit Fluid Volume (Dehydration)
    Orthostatic Hypotension (Postural Hypotension)

Basic Life Support by Health-Care Providers (Cardiopulmonary Resuscitation, CPR)

Definition: External cardiac compression and ventilation to ↑blood flow to heart and brain; follows sequence of circulation, airway, breathing (CAB).

1. Shake shoulder and shout, "Are you OK?" Assesses level of consciousness.
2. If no response, call for help or activate the emergency medical services (EMS) system; ensures help and presence of defibrillator and resuscitative medications.
3. Palpate carotid pulse for adult or brachial/femoral pulse for infant/child; assesses circulation.
4. Deliver 30 external cardiac compressions; promotes cardiac output (ensure victim is on hard surface in supine position).

CPR	Infant (<1 yr)	Child (>1 yr–adolescent)	Adult
Rate of compressions.	At least 100 compressions per minute. Rotate health-care provider every 2 min; interruptions less than 10 seconds.		
Compression landmark.	Center of chest below nipples.	Center of chest between nipples.	Lower half of sternum.
Depth of compressions.	⅓ of anteroposterior (AP) diameter. About 1.5 inches.	⅓ of AP diameter. About 2 inches.	At least 2 inches.

Continued

CPR	Infant (<1 yr)	Child (>1 yr–adolescent)	Adult
Ratio of compressions to ventilations.	30 to 2 (one rescuer). 15 to 2 (two rescuers).		30 to 2 (one or two rescuers).
Compression method "hard and fast" with complete chest recoil.	Two fingers (one rescuer). Two thumbs with hands encircling chest (two rescuers).	Heel of one hand. *or* Heel of one hand with fingers interlocked with the other.	Heel of one hand with fingers interlocked with the other.

5. Assess and establish airway; open airway (head-tilt, chin-lift maneuver or jaw thrust without neck hyperextension if cervical injury suspected); listen, look, and feel for air exchange.
6. If not breathing, give two breaths; instill air into lungs (maintain head-tilt or jaw thrust maneuver while pinching victim's nostrils).
7. Maintain ratio of compressions to ventilations for five cycles and then reassess pulse.
8. Defibrillate; minimize length of interruptions.
9. If successful, discontinue CPR and position victim in recovery position.
10. If unsuccessful, resume compressions and then ventilations according to appropriate age and number of rescuer's ratio; terminate CPR when ordered by primary health-care provider or rescuer exhaustion.

Foreign Body Airway Obstruction

	Infant (<1 yr)	Child (>1 yr–adolescent)	Adult
Assess Extent of Obstruction	**Partial:** Can cough and make sounds. **Total:** Cannot cough, make sounds, or speak; difficulty breathing; pallor; cyanosis.		**Partial:** Can cough and make sounds. **Total:** Hands encircle throat (universal choking sign); ask "Are you choking?"

Foreign Body Airway Obstruction—cont'd

	Infant (<1 yr)	Child (>1 yr–adolescent)	Adult
Victim Is Conscious	**Partial:** Monitor; allow victim's efforts to dislodge object.		
	Total: Deliver five back blows and five chest thrusts; repeat until object is expelled or victim is unresponsive.	**Total:** Activate EMS system; ask "Can I help?" • Initiate abdominal thrust maneuver: Encircle conscious victim's waist and with intertwined clenched fists, thrust upward and inward against diaphragm. • Deliver abdominal thrusts until object is expelled or victim is unresponsive.	
Victim Is Unconscious	Head-tilt, chin-lift maneuver; inspect mouth; remove object if present in pharynx; implement CPR but inspect mouth before each two rescue breaths.		

Ethical and Legal Foundations

Basics of Ethical Decision Making

- **Patient Care Partnership** (American Hospital Association): Information about what patients should expect about their rights and responsibilities when hospitalized, including high-quality hospital care, clean and safe environment, involvement in care, protection of privacy, and help when leaving the hospital and with billing. www.aha.org/aha/issues/Communicating-With-Patients/pt-care-partnership.html
- **Autonomy:** Support personal freedom and decision making.
- **Beneficence:** Promote good.
- **Fidelity:** Keep promises and commitments.
- **Justice:** Treat people fairly and equally.
- **Nonmaleficence:** Do no harm.
- **Paternalism:** Make or allow a person to make a decision for another.
- **Respect:** Acknowledge rights of others.
- **Veracity:** Tell the truth.

Legal Terms

- **Advance directive:** Written document that addresses treatment desires in the future if unable to make decisions.
- **Living will:** Specifically identifies treatment desires.
- **Health-care proxy** (durable power of attorney): Assigns decision making to another.
- **Do not resuscitate:** Order stating that a patient should not be revived; at request of patient when able; health-care proxy, family member, or legal guardian when patient is unable to give consent.
- **Assault:** Threat of unlawful touching of another.
- **Battery:** Unlawful touching of another without consent, such as procedures performed without consent.
- **False imprisonment:** Restriction/retention of patient without consent; use restraints in compliance with policy and procedure; have patient sign release if desiring to leave facility against medical advice.
- **Good Samaritan law:** Legal protection for those who render care in an emergency without expectation of remuneration.
- **Libel:** Written statement causing harm to patient.
- **Malpractice:** Professional negligence; for example, when the nurse owed a duty to the patient but did not carry out that duty, and it resulted in injury to the patient.
- **Negligence:** Failing to perform an act that a reasonable prudent nurse would do under similar circumstances; may be an act of omission or commission. Examples: Failure to ensure patient safety (falls); improper performance of a treatment (burns from warm soak); medication errors; inappropriate use of equipment (excessive IVF via pump); and failure to assess, report, or document a patient's status.
- **Organ donation:** Donor card, living will, or family consent if patient is unable to participate in decision is necesary to donate organs.
- **Respondeat superior:** Latin term meaning "let the master answer"; employer is responsible for acts of employees causing harm during employment activities.
- **Slander:** Oral statement resulting in damage to a patient; for example, nurse incorrectly tells others that a patient has AIDS and it affects the patient's business.
- **Uniform Determination of Death Act:**
- **Cardiopulmonary criteria:** Irreversible cessation of circulatory and respiratory function.
- **Whole-brain criteria:** Irreversible cessation of all functions of the entire brain and brain stem; organs may be healthy for donation even though meeting whole-brain criteria.

Disease and Treatment Mnemonics

CAUTION: Early Signs of Cancer	INFECT: S&S of Infection
Change in bowel or bladder habits. **A** sore throat that does not heal. **U**nusual bleeding or discharge. **T**hickening or lump. **I**ndigestion; dysphagia. **O**bvious change in a wart or mole. **N**agging cough or hoarseness.	**I**ncreased pulse, respirations, white blood cells (WBCs). **N**odes are enlarged. **F**unction is impaired. **E**rythema, edema, exudate. **C**omplains of discomfort or pain. **T**emperature—local or systemic.

Treatment for Acute Injury

Rest: Decreases stress/strain on injury.
Ice: Vasoconstriction decreases edema and pain.
Compression: External pressure decreases edema and pain.
Elevate: Gravity decreases edema.

Phases of the Therapeutic Nurse-Patient Relationship

Phase	Nurse	Patient
Preinteraction: Begins before patient contact.	• Explore personal feelings, values, attitudes. • Collect data about patient. • Plan for first interaction.	• Has no role in this phase.
Orientation: Introductory phase; begins at first meeting.	• Listen; be empathetic. • Identify boundaries of relationship (termination begins here). • Clarify expectations. • Establish rapport.	• Recognize need for help. • Commit to a therapeutic relationship. • Begin to test relationship.
Working: Begins when patient identifies problems to be worked on.	• Assist with exploration of issues. • Support healthy problem solving.	• Develop trust in nurse. • Examine personal issues. • Develop strategies to resolve issues.

Continued

Phases of the Therapeutic Nurse-Patient Relationship—cont'd

Phase	Nurse	Patient
	• Assist with strategy development. • Identify own reactions to patient based on own needs, conflicts, relationships **(counter-transference).**	• May superimpose feelings from another relationship onto the nurse-patient relationship **(transference).**
Resolution: Termination phase; begins when problems are resolved and ends when relationship is terminated.	• Review goals and objectives achieved. • Reinforce adaptive behaviors. • Share feelings about termination. • Avoid discussing previous or new issues. • Encourage independence; focus on future. • Promote positive family interactions. • Refer to community resources.	• Share feelings about termination (anger, rejection, regression; negative feelings may be expressed to deal with loss). • May attempt to discuss previous or new issues. • Assume responsibility for use of community resources.

Interviewing

Interviewing Skills

■ **Active listening:** Absorbs content and patient's feelings; uses all senses. *Nurse*: verbal/nonverbal attending, appropriate gestures (head nodding), eye contact, sitting, open posture, vocal cues ("mmm").

■ **Clarification:** Asks for more information; checks accuracy; ↓ ambiguity. *Nurse*: "I am not sure I know what you mean by that."

■ **Confrontation:** Presents reality; identifies inconsistencies; ↑ self-awareness; use gently after trust is developed. *Patient*: "I never have any visitors." *Nurse*: "I was here yesterday when you had three visitors."

■ **Direct:** Collects specific information quickly. *Nurse*: "Where is your pain?"

- **Focusing:** Let patient finish thoughts; centers on key elements to ↓ rambling. *Nurse*: "When talking about your house, you mentioned scatter rugs. Let's talk more about being safe in your home."
- **Nonverbal:** Promotes verbalization. *Nurse*: Lean forward, nod head, smile, use gestures.
- **Open-ended:** Invites elaboration; nonthreatening; avoids yes and no answers. *Nurse*: "Tell me about what a typical day is like for you."
- **Paraphrasing:** Restates message in similar words; focuses on content; encourages discussion. *Patient*: "I may not make it." *Nurse*: "You think you are going to die?"
- **Reflection:** Describes or interprets feelings or mood. *Nurse*: "You sound upset."
- **Silence:** Allows for reflection and patient response; prompts talking; useful when patient is sad or remaining quiet.
- **Summarizing:** Reviews key elements; brings closure; clarifies expectations. *Nurse*: "Today we talked about . . ."
- **Touch:** Conveys caring; is reassuring; may invade personal space. *Nurse*: hold patient's hand, gently pat patient's shoulder, avoid touching suspicious, paranoic, or angry patients.
- **Validation:** Confirms what the nurse heard or observed. *Nurse*: "I understand that you just said . . ."

Barriers to Communication

- Pain
- Advising
- Changing topic
- Failing to listen
- Trite, common expressions (clichés)
- Judgmental or minimizing comments
- Direct probing and "how" and "why" questions
- Overly optimistic statements (false reassurance)
- Challenging, defensive, or disapproving responses
- Interruptions, environmental noise, or extremes in temperature

Leadership and Management

Leadership and Management Terms

- **Accountability:** Answerable for actions and judgments regarding care.
- **Autonomy:** Nurse can make independent decision to act.
- **Case management:** Coordination of interdisciplinary care for patient.
- **Decentralized management:** Staff participates in decision making.

- **Performance appraisal:** Evaluation of a nurse's compliance (quality and quantity) with standards and roles within job description.
- **Professional standards:** Actions consistent with minimum safe professional conduct. Description of responsibilities (American Nurses Association, Joint Commission, agency policy and procedure).
- **Quality improvement:** Activities to ↑ achievement of ideal care.
- **Responsibility:** Duties and activities the nurse is hired to perform.

Leadership Styles

- **Autocratic:** Complete control over decisions, goals, plans, and evaluation of outcomes; firm, insistent; often used in emergencies or when staff is inexperienced or new.
- **Democratic:** Participative; shares responsibilities; uses role to motivate staff to achieve communal goals **(shared governance)**; encourages intercommunication and contributions; used to help staff grow in abilities; ↑ motivation; ↑ staff satisfaction.
- **Laissez-faire:** Nondirective; relinquishes control and direction to staff; best used with experienced, expert, mature staff who know roles.
- **Transformational:** Presents vision for the future, provides supportive climate, acts as coach or mentor, inspires commitment to the good of the group, promotes creativity; best used in self-governing situations.

Leader Qualities

Effective leaders and managers need to:
Understand human behavior.

- Have insight into its relationship to beliefs, values, feelings.
- Be sensitive to others' feelings and problems.

Use effective communication skills.

- Be clear, concise, avoid ambiguity.
- Use appropriate format (verbal, written, formal, informal).
- Be aware of own nonverbal behavior.

Use power appropriately.

- Use power attained through place in table of organization (positional). Do not abuse power.
- Use power attained through knowledge and experience or perceived by staff (professional).

Respond to staff needs.

- Listen attentively; attend to needs; provide positive feedback; avoid favoritism; set realistic expectations; avoid mixed messages.

- Treat staff with respect; counsel privately; keep promises; avoid threats, superior attitude, criticism, or aggressive confrontation.

Delegate appropriately (leader retains accountability).

- Right person (competent subordinate).
- Right task (within scope of practice).
- Right situation (appropriate to abilities and patient acuity).
- Right communication (clear instructions, validate understanding).
- Right supervision (assess actions, evaluate outcomes).

Provide opportunities for personal growth.

- Help less-experienced nurse to ↑ knowledge, experience, responsibility (mentor/preceptor, continuing education, staff education).

Use critical thinking and problem solving.

- Encourage staff to engage in critical thinking by involving in assessing, planning, and evaluating outcomes.

Recognize and address conditions conducive to change.

- Ensure that all staff have a stake in the outcome; include all creatively in the process; focus on benefits; provide positive feedback; offer incentives.
- Ensure change is planned, introduced gradually, initiated in a calm rather than chaotic atmosphere; best after a prior successful change.
- Recognize and address resistance; identify causes of resistance: threatening; lack of understanding; disagreeing with purpose/approach, beliefs, values; ↑ in responsibility; content with status quo; fear of failure.

Levels of Management

First level: Supervises nonmanagerial staff; oversees day-to-day activities of a group (team leader, charge nurse).
Middle level: Supervises a group of first-level managers (supervisor, coordinator).
Upper level: Organizational executives; sets goals and strategic planning (VP for nursing, associate director of nursing).

Nurse Manager Role

- Functions as a role model regarding professional conduct.
- Sets standards of performance; establishes goals for the unit with the staff; mobilizes staff and agency resources to attain goals.
- Supports mutual trust; treats staff with respect; counsels privately.
- Empowers staff; supports innovation; seeks staff members' opinions; promotes professional environment and growth; rewards growth.
- Performs patient rounds with multidisciplinary team.

- Evaluates nursing practice and achievement of standards.
- Designs and implements a quality improvement (QI) program for the unit; engages staff in QI activities.
- Assists in staff development plan and orientation of new employees.
- Schedules staffing for unit; conducts staff meetings with all shifts.
- Evaluates performance of subordinates (performance appraisal).
- Participates in intradepartmental and interdepartmental meetings.

Staff Nurse Role

- Functions as role model regarding professional conduct.
- Receives report from and makes rounds with nurse previously responsible for patient.
- Assesses, analyzes, and interprets data; identifies nursing diagnoses; formulates a plan of care; evaluates patient responses to care and extent of outcome achievement.
- Sets priorities regarding patient needs; progresses from those who have an immediate threat to survival (problems with breathing, vital signs, ↓ level of consciousness); to requests for help (pain, toileting); to important but not immediate needs (teaching).
- Coordinates and/or performs care for assigned patients; uses time-management skills; completes all care assigned.
- Performs professional procedures such as sterile irrigations, insertion of a urinary catheter, colostomy irrigation, tracheal suctioning, administering medication and parenteral therapies, patient teaching.
- Delegates care to subordinates that is within their job description.
- Evaluates care delegated; establishes clear expectations; encourages communication; evaluates patient outcomes related to delegated tasks (nurse retains accountability for delegated tasks).
- Gives report to next nurse responsible for patient.
- Engages in QI activities.
- Participates in intradepartmental and interdepartmental meetings.

Unlicensed Assistive Personnel Role

- Works within scope of practice determined by agency policy; performs activities with established sequence of steps with little or no modification and reasonable predictable results; provides direct care for only stable patients.
- Cannot engage in activities outside their role; pervasive functions of assessment, planning, evaluation, and nursing judgment cannot be delegated (NCSBN 2005); examples: performing a physical assessment, formulating plans of care, teaching, implementing complex tasks, caring for unstable patients.

- Obtains vital signs.
- Performs hygiene and comfort activities (bathing, backrub).
- Assists patients with ADLs such as eating, drinking, toileting (bedpan, commode), ambulation (walking, transfer).
- Changes linens.
- Empties urinary retention collection device.
- Transports patients.

Community Nursing

- **Community health nursing (public health nursing):** Nursing care for a specific population living in the same geographic area, or groups having similar values, interests, needs; aims to develop a healthy environment in which to live.
- **Public health functions:** Community assessment, policy development, facilitating access to resources; cohesiveness is promoted by engaging community members in the problem solving process and promoting empowerment through education, opportunities, resources; successful public health programs are congruent with that of the interests and goals of the community.
- **Assessment of a community:**
  - **Structure (milieu):** Geographical area, environment, housing, economy, water, sanitation.
  - **Population:** Age and sex distribution, density, growth trends, educational level, cultures and subcultures, religious groups.
  - **Social systems:** Education, communication, transportation, welfare, health-care delivery systems (governmental, voluntary agencies).
- **Community-based nursing:** Nursing care delivered in the community while focused on a specific individual's or family's health-care needs; individual viewed within the larger systems of family, community, culture, society.
- **Vulnerable populations:** Homeless, living in poverty, migrant workers, living in rural communities, pregnant adolescents, suicidal individuals, frail older adults.
- **Stigmatized groups:** People viewed with disdain because of a disease or behavior (HIV, substance abuse, mental illness).
- **Settings in which nurses work:** Homes, community health centers, clinics, industry, rehabilitation centers, schools, crisis intervention centers and phone lines, shelters, halfway houses, sheltered workshops, day-care centers, forensic settings.
- **Roles of nurses:** Discharge planner, case manager, counselor, health promoter, case finder, caregiver, educator, researcher, consultant, advocate, role model, change agent.
- **Hospice care:** Supportive care (**palliative**) for dying persons and their caregivers usually during last 6 month of life; experts in pain and symptom

management; focuses on preserving dignity and quality of life; supports bereavement.
- **Respite care:** Temporary care for the homebound so caregivers have relief from day-to-day responsibilities.

Patient Education

Learning Domains

Cognitive
- Thinking, acquiring, comprehending, synthesizing, evaluating, storing, recalling information.
- Builds on what patient knows; presents essential information first; adds information as patient asks questions.
- Teaching strategies: Lecture, discussion, audiovisuals, printed material, computer-assisted instruction, Web-based instruction.
- Evaluation: Assesses knowledge by verbal and written means.

Affective
- Addresses attitudes, feelings, beliefs, values.
- Recognizes that it takes patient time to internalize need-to-change behavior.
- Understands own value system; respects uniqueness of each patient; helps patient explore feelings.
- Teaching strategies: Discussion, play, role-modeling, panel discussion, groups, role-playing.
- Evaluation: Evidence of behavior incorporated into lifestyle.

Psychomotor
- Addresses physical and motor skills; requires dexterity and coordination to manipulate equipment; ultimately performs a task with skill.
- Ensures mastery of each step before moving to next step.
- Teaching strategies: Audiovisuals, pictures, demonstrations, models.
- Evaluation: Observation of performance of skill (return demonstration).

Teaching and Learning: General Concepts
- Education can prevent illness; promote or restore health; ↑ complications; ↓ independence and coping; ↑ individual and family growth; incorporate throughout health-care delivery.
- Environment should be conducive to learning: private, quiet, well lit, comfortable, lacking distractions (close doors and curtains; shut off TV).
- Teaching process should follow format of the nursing process (assessment, analysis, planning, implementation, and evaluation).

- Both short- and long-term goals should be set to ↑ motivation and allow for evaluation; goals must be patient centered, specific, measurable, realistic, have a time frame.
- A variety of teaching strategies that use different senses should be used (written materials, videos, discussion, demonstration).
- Teaching can be formal or informal, individualized or within a group.
- Information should move from simple to complex, from known to unknown, and be appropriate for patient's cognitive and developmental levels.
- Shorter, more frequent sessions are most effective (15–30 min).
- Learning is ↑ with repetition, consistency, practice.
- Evaluation and documentation are essential elements of teaching.

Patient Factors That Influence Learning

Culture, Religion, Ethnicity, Language
Commonalities and differences exist between cultures and among people from within the same culture.

Nursing Care
- Be culturally sensitive and nonjudgmental.
- Avoid assumptions, biases, stereotypes; seek help from multicultural team.
- Provide teaching in patient's language; use professional translator.

Knowledge and Experience
Can promote or deter learning.

Nursing Care
- Identify what patient already knows; build on this foundation.
- Explore concerns related to experiences; correct misconceptions.

Literacy
Years in school may not accurately reflect reading ability.

Nursing Care
- Assess ability to read, comprehend material (confusion, nervousness, excuses may indicate ↓ ability to read).
- Use illustrations, models, videos, discussion.
- Provide privacy.

Developmental Level
- **Children:** The younger the child, the shorter the attention span; may regress developmentally when ill; imagination can ↑ fear and misconceptions; toddlers and preschoolers are concrete thinkers; school-age children are capable of logical thinking.

Nursing Care

- Identify developmental age to determine appropriate strategies (dolls, puppets, role-playing, drawing, games, books).
- Use direct, simple approach.
- Include parents.

Adolescents: Need to be similar to peers; seek autonomy; focus on the present.

Nursing Care

- Be open and honest about the illness.
- Respect opinions and need to be like peers.
- Support need for control.
- Ensure learning has immediate results.

Adults: Need to be self-sufficient and in control; learning most effective when self-directed.

Nursing Care

- Assess for readiness; explore perceived benefit.
- Built on prior knowledge and experience.

Older adults: Needs are highly variable; functional changes, stress, fatigue, chronic illness can ↑ learning; changes may include slower cognition and reaction time, becoming overwhelmed with too much detail, ↑ ability to recall new information.

Nursing Care

- Do not underestimate learning ability.
- Plan shorter, more frequent teaching sessions.
- Decrease pace of teaching to allow more time to process information, make decisions.
- Teach main points and avoid irrelevant details.

Readiness to Learn: Receptiveness to Learning

Patient has to recognize need to learn and be physically and emotionally able to participate.

Nursing Care

- Identify readiness: Patient states misconceptions, asks questions, demonstrates health-seeking behaviors, is physically comfortable, and anxiety is less than moderate.
- Identify physical adaptations that may interfere with learning: pain, acute or chronic illness, oxygen deprivation, fatigue, weakness, and sensory impairment.
- Identify emotional and mental adaptations that interfere with learning: anxiety, anger, denial, and impaired cognition.
- Select teaching aids appropriate for patient's sensory limitations (↓ sight, ↑ hearing).

- Postpone teaching until patient is able to focus on learning; address factors that interfere with learning.

Motivation
Motivation is the drive that causes action; essential to learning.

Nursing Care
- Identify the patient's personal desire to learn (intrinsic motivation, internal locus of control).
- Identify the patient's desire to learn because of an external reward (extrinsic motivation, external locus of control).
- Be sincere and nonjudgmental.
- Ensure material is meaningful; make contractual agreement; set short-term goals to ensure success.
- Identify and praise progress (positive reinforcement); avoid criticism (negative reinforcement); allow for mistakes.
- Assess for ↓ motivation (distraction, changing subject).

Infection Control

Standard Precautions: Tier 1

- Perform hand hygiene before and after care and when soiled; most important way to prevent infection.
- Use personal protective equipment (PPE) if touching, spilling, or splashing of blood or body fluids is likely; use gloves, gowns, mask, goggles, face shield, aprons, head and foot protection.
- Discard disposable items in fluid-impermeable bag and contaminated items in biohazard red bag.
- Dispose sharps in a sharps container; do not recap used needles.
- Hold linen away from body; place linen in fluid-impermeable bag in a covered hamper; do not let hampers overflow.
- Place lab specimens in a leak-proof transport bag without contaminating the outside; label with biohazard sticker and patient information.
- Institute procedure for accidental exposure: Wash area, report to supervisor, receive emergency care, seek referral for follow-up.
- Receive hepatitis B vaccine.
- Assign patient to private room if hygiene practices are unacceptable.
- Avoid eating, drinking, touching eyes, applying makeup in patient areas.

Transmission-Based Precautions: Tier 2

Airborne

- Used for microorganisms that spread through air (droplet nuclei <5 μm) such as TB, measles, chickenpox.
- Private room; negative air pressure room; door closed; high-efficiency disposable mask (replace when moist) or particulate respirator such as for TB; mask on patient when transporting; teach to dispose soiled tissues in fluid-impervious bag at bedside.

Droplet

- Used for microorganisms spread by large-particle droplets (droplet nuclei >5 μm) such as pneumonia (streptococcal, mycoplasmal, meningococcal), rubella, mumps, influenza, adenovirus.
- Private room if available or cohort patients; wear mask when within 3 feet of patient; may keep door open; mask on patient when transporting; teach patient to dispose soiled tissues in fluid-impervious bag at bedside.

Contact

- Used for microorganisms spread by direct or indirect contact such as methicillin-resistant *S. aureus* (MRSA), vancomycin-resistant enterococcus (VRE), vancomycin intermediate-resistant *S. aureus* (VISA), enteric pathogens (*E. coli, C. difficile*), herpes simplex, pediculosis, hepatitis A and E, varicella zoster, respiratory syncytial virus.
- Private room or cohort patients; gown; position gloves over gown cuffs; dedicated equipment.

Neutropenic Precautions

- For individuals with compromised immune system.
- Use standard precautions, especially hand hygiene.
- Caregivers and visitors should be free of communicable illnesses.
- Private room if possible; keep room meticulously clean.
- Teach to avoid sources of potential infection such as crowds, confined spaces (airplane, theaters), raw fruits and vegetables, flowers and plants.

Surgical (Sterile) Asepsis

- Check expiration date; ensure packages are dry, intact, stain-free.
- Discard opened sterile solutions older than 24 hr; criteria for medicated and antiseptic solutions may differ.
- Place cap on table with inner cap turned up; label with date, time, initials; avoid touching bottle rim.
- Place sterile equipment inside the outer 1 inch of sterile field.

- Ensure that sterile objects touch only another sterile object.
- Open sterile packages away from sterile field.
- Keep sterile field in line of vision.
- Position solution closest to patient; keep field dry and free of moisture.
- Don sterile gloves without contaminating sterile surfaces.
- Keep sterile gloved hands and equipment above level of waist.
- Avoid talking, coughing, sneezing around a sterile field.
- Discard sterile objects that become contaminated or if in doubt.

Basic Nursing Measures

Body Mechanics

- Follow principles of body mechanics and maintain functional alignment: ↑ balance, movement, physiological function; avoid stress on muscles, tendons, ligaments, bones, joints; avoid rotating or twisting body; use supportive devices.
- Keep weight within the center of gravity; avoid reaching.
- Spread feet apart to widen base of support.
- Use large muscles of legs for power.
- Flex knees and hold objects being lifted close to body (lowers center of gravity and keeps weight within base of support).
- Raise bed to working height; transfer patient from higher surface to lower surface (uses gravity).
- Use internal girdle to stabilize pelvis when lifting, pulling, stooping.
- Use body weight as a force for pushing and pulling; lean forward and backward or rock on feet.
- Pull, push, roll, slide rather than lift; face direction of movement.

Fall Prevention

- Assess for risk factors: history of falls; ↓ sensory perception; weakness; ↓ mobility; ↓ LOC; ↓ mental capacity; ↑ anxiety; confusion; medications (diuretics, opioids, antihypertensives).
- Orient to bed and room; teach use of ambulatory aids and call bell; answer call bell immediately.
- Keep bed in lowest position unless receiving care.
- Raise three of four side rails; raise four rails if it is patient's preference or if there is an order (four raised rails are considered a restraint).
- Lock wheels on all equipment; ensure that equipment is intact.
- Keep call bell, bedside and overbed table, personal items in reach.
- Keep floor dry and free of electric cords and obstacles; use night-light.
- Encourage use of grab bars, railings, rubber-soled shoes.

- Stay with patient in bathroom or shower (need order for shower).
- Teach fall-prevention techniques such as rising slowly.
- Use monitoring device that will alert the nurse if a patient attempts to ambulate unassisted.

Fire Safety

- Stay calm; keep halls clear; do not use elevator; stay close to the floor (smoke rises).
- Know location, use of alarms and extinguishers.
- Evacuate patients in immediate danger first and then ambulatory, those needing assistance, and finally bedbound patients.
- **Class A fire:** Wood, textiles, paper trash; use water extinguisher.
- **Class B fire:** Oil, grease, paint, chemicals; use dry powder and CO_2 extinguisher (water will spread fire); avoid touching horn of CO_2 extinguisher because it can freeze tissue.
- **Class C fire:** Electrical wires, appliances, motors; use dry powder or CO_2 extinguisher (water will cause electrocution).
- **RACE: R**escue patients in danger; **A**ctivate alarm; **C**ontain fire (close doors and windows); **E**xtinguish fire if small; **E**vacuate horizontally and then vertically.

Pain Management

Pain Rating Scales

FACES Pain Rating Scale

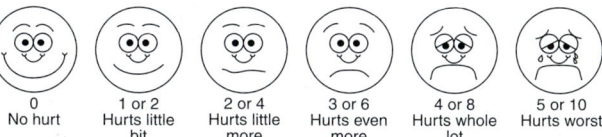

0	1 or 2	2 or 4	3 or 6	4 or 8	5 or 10
No hurt	Hurts little bit	Hurts little more	Hurts even more	Hurts whole lot	Hurts worst

Source: Wong-Baker FACES Pain Rating Scale. From Hockenberry-Eaton M., Willson D. Wong's Nursing Care of Infants and Children, 8th ed. St. Louis, MO, 2007, p. 210. Copyrighted by Mosby. Reprinted by permission.

PQRST Pain Rating Scale

P: Provokes/point: What causes the pain? Point to the pain.
Q: Quality: Is it dull, achy, sharp, stabbing, pressuring, deep, etc.?
R: Radiation/relief: Does it radiate? What makes it better or worse?

S: Severity/signs and symptoms (S&S): Rate pain on 0–10 scale. What S&S are associated with the pain such as dizziness, diaphoresis, dyspnea, abnormal VS?

T: Time/onset: When did it start? Is it constant or intermittent? How long does it last? Sudden or gradual onset? Frequency?

Nursing Care for Patients in Pain

- **Assess pain:** Presence, severity, characteristics (see pain rating scales, p. 32).
- **Validate patient's pain:** Accept that pain exists.
- **Provide comfort:** Positioning, rest.
- **Relieve anxiety:** Answer questions, provide emotional support.
- **Teach relaxation techniques:** Rhythmic breathing, guided imagery.
- **Provide cutaneous stimulation:** Backrub, heat and cold therapy.
- **Decrease irritating stimuli:** Bright lights, noise, ↑↓ room temperature.
- **Use distraction for mild pain:** Music, TV, reading, imagery.
- **Give prescribed medications:** Analgesics, opioids, antispasmodics.
- **Evaluate patient response:** Document, modify plan.

Nursing Care for Patients in Restraints

Introduction
- Physical or chemical intervention that ↓ movement.
- Purpose: Preventing falls, disrupting therapy, harming self or others.
- Physical restraints: Devices used to ↓ movement, such as vest, mitt, wrist, elbow, belt, mummy.
- Chemical restraints: Medications to calm disruptive or combative behavior that may cause harm to self or others.

Nursing Care
- Document behavior requiring need and failure of less invasive measures to protect patient.
- In an emergency, obtain order from primary health-care provider and additional order per agency and state policies.
- Ensure functional alignment before applying.
- Follow directions (correct size, snug but does not limit respirations or occlude circulation, apply vest with V opening in front).
- Pad under wrist when using wrist or mitt restraints.
- Secure straps with slipknot to bed frame.
- Assess respiratory and circulatory status routinely.
- Every 1–2 hours remove restraint, assess skin, massage area, perform ROM.

Nursing Care for Patients With Visual Impairments

- Knock on door; greet patient by name; identify self; explain purpose.
- Do not touch until patient understands your name and purpose.
- Approach in an unhurried manner; use clear, simple sentences.
- Stay within patient's field of vision; approach from strong side.
- Orient to room, location; use of call bell.
- Provide a predictable environment; remove all hazards.
- Limit noise and distraction in environment; explain unusual noises.
- Ensure eyeglasses are clean, accessible, and protected when stored.
- Inform of location of food on meal tray; use numbers on a clock.
- Ambulate patient by walking slightly in front while patient holds your arm; never try to push or guide from behind; inform of doors, steps.
- Make it clear to patient when conversation is over or when leaving area.

Nursing Care for Patients With Hearing Impairments

- Greet patient by name; identify yourself and your purpose; ↓ environmental noise when communicating.
- Use touch appropriately to alert patient that you are about to talk.
- Face patient directly; avoid turning away from patient while you are speaking; avoid covering your mouth with your hand to facilitate lipreading.
- Talk in a normal tone at a moderate rate; speak clearly; articulate consonants carefully; do not overly articulate or yell.
- Use gestures and facial expressions to convey message.
- Encourage use of hearing aid; facilitate repair of nonworking aids.
- Remove hearing aid when showering or washing hair.
- Follow manufacturer's directions to insert, remove, clean, store aid.

Nursing Care for Patients With a Latex Allergy

Type of Reaction	S&S	Nursing Care
• **Local skin reaction**: Direct skin-to-latex contact. • Excessive exposure can lead to systemic reaction.	• Not life-threatening. • Erythema, pruritus, popular, vesicular, scaling, or bleeding lesions.	• Apply allergy wristband. • Label chart. • Use latex-free equipment such as gloves, tape, dressings, syringes, antiembolism stockings, tubing, tourniquets, stethoscopes, electrode pads, BP cuffs, indwelling urinary catheters.
• **Systemic**: Direct skin-to-latex contact. • Contact with equipment exposed to latex.	• Life-threatening. • Angioedema. • Rhinitis or rhinorrhea. • Conjunctivitis. • Bronchospasm.	
• Powder particles exposed to latex may be inhaled or absorbed via skin, mucous membranes, or blood.	• Anaphylactic responses. • Circulatory collapse.	• Notify pharmacy so meds and mixed solutions are latex-free. • Ensure procedure rooms are latex-free and patient is first case of the day.

Nursing Care of Older Adults (>65 Yr)

Demographic Data
About 70% rate themselves as healthy; majority live in the community; increasingly more live in independent or assisted-living communities; 5% in nursing homes.

Physical Changes
Gradual ↓ in physical abilities; close vision impairment (presbyopia); ↓ hearing, especially for high-pitched sounds; ↓ subcutaneous tissue; ↓ muscle strength; ↓ balance and coordination; ↓ immune response; one or more chronic health problems.

Psychosocial Issues
Conflict is ego integrity vs. despair; reminisces about past; personality does not change but may become exaggerated; adjusting to aging, ↓ health, quality of life,

retirement, fixed income, death of spouse or friends, change in residence, own mortality; may become focused on bodily needs and comforts; sexual expression (love, touching, sharing, intercourse) important and related to identity.

Cognitive Status
IQ does not ↓; mental acuity slows (↑ time to learn and problem solve); long-term memory better than short-term memory.

Reaction to Illness and Hospitalization
Illness and recuperation longer due to ↓ adaptive capacity; ↑ feelings of inadequacy and mortality; may ↑ self-absorption, social isolation, frustration, anger, depression, especially if retirement goals are denied; unfamiliar environment may cause confusion, anxiety; chronic illness, pain, or impending death may cause dependence, hopelessness; may accept and prepare for death.

General Nursing Care
- Understand commonalities of aging, but approach each person as unique.
- Avoid stereotyping because it denies uniqueness; ↓ access to care impacts negatively on individual.
- Ensure access to health care and social services, especially in home; critical illnesses deserve aggressive treatment, if desired.

Common Problems Associated With Aging

Bowel and Bladder Incontinence
Not part of aging process; may be aggravated by ↓ muscle tone of anal and urinary sphincters and prostatic hypertrophy.

- **Nursing care:** Ensure screening for urinary tract infection (UTI), bladder and prostate cancer; assist with hygiene and skin care; institute bowel or bladder retraining.

Adverse Drug Effects
Multiple health problems require ↑ prescriptions (**polypharmacy**) with ↓ coordination among primary health-care providers; ↓ hepatic and renal function results in drug accumulation; ↑ paradoxical drug effects.

- **Nursing care:** ↑ coordination of health care; identify unnecessary or excessive doses of medications; assess for adverse and toxic effects.

Falls and Accidents
Occur due to sensory impairments (vision, hearing, sensation), postural changes, ↓ muscle strength and endurance, orthostatic hypotension, neurological and cardiovascular decline.
- **Nursing care:** Assist with ambulation; teach safety precautions such as use of grab bars, railings, walker; rise slowly; keep feet apart for a wide base; give up driving when impairment jeopardizes safety.

Infection
Increased risk due to ↓ immune response.

- **Nursing care:** Teach preventive measures such as hand hygiene, avoiding crowds, smoking cessation; give prescribed pneumonia vaccine and yearly flu vaccine.

Cognitive Impairment
Not part of aging process.
Delirium is an acute, reversible state of agitated confusion.
Dementia is a chronic, progressive, irreversible disorder.
Sundowning syndrome is confusion beginning in late afternoon or evening.

- **Nursing care:** See Tab 5, MENTAL HEALTH, Nursing Care for Patients With Dementia or Decreased Cognition, p. 165.

Alcohol Abuse
Associated with depression, loneliness, lack of social support.

- **Nursing care:** Explore effective coping strategies; refer to AA.

Risk of Dehydration
Occurs due to ↓ thirst mechanism; ↓ ability to concentrate urine; med side effects.

- **Nursing care:** Encourage intake of at least 1.5–2 L fluid daily; teach to seek care if vomiting or diarrhea occurs >24 hours.

Risk of Suicide
Associated with multiple losses (loved ones, health); lack of social support; depression; feelings of hopelessness; isolation.

- **Nursing care:** Assess for suicide risk; provide reality orientation; validation therapy; reminiscence; support body image; encourage psychological counseling; obtain prescription for antidepressant; refer to social service agency.

Sexual Responsiveness/Erectile Dysfunction
Sexual response takes longer related to ↓ estrogen and testosterone, chronic health problems, and drug side effect; unavailable partner; cognitive impairment.

- **Nursing care:** Provide for privacy and dignity; maintain nonjudgmental attitude; ↑ verbalization of concerns; suggest use of lubricants, penile prostheses, medications to increase erectile function.

Sexually Transmitted Infections (STIs)
Need for sexual expression continues; ↑ society recognition that sex is natural and acceptable even if single by choice or death of spouse.

- **Nursing care:** Maintain nonjudgmental attitude; teach about STI prevention.

Leading Causes of Death

Heart disease, then cancer, stroke, lung disease, falls, diabetes, kidney and liver disease; often have one or more chronic illnesses.

■ **Nursing care:** Focus on health promotion; encourage smoking cessation, ↑ exercise, weight control, adequate nutrition; provide screening programs to identify problems early; encourage health-care supervision to manage chronic conditions.

Common Human Responses and Related Nursing Care

Vital Signs

Temperature

Afebrile
- ■ **Oral:** 97.5°F–99.5°F
- ■ **Rectal:** 0.5°F–1°F more than oral route

Hyperthermia: >99.5°F
Hypothermia: <97.5°F

Pulse

Normal: 60–100 bpm
Tachycardia: >100 bpm
Bradycardia: <60 bpm
Thready: Weak, feeble
Bounding: Forceful, full
Dysrhythmia: Irregular pattern
Pulse deficit: Difference between radial and apical rate

Respirations

Eupnea: Expected rate 12–20 bpm
Tachypnea: >20 bpm
Bradypnea: <12 bpm
Apnea: Absence of breathing
Hyperventilation: ↑ rate and depth
Hypoventilation: ↓ rate and depth
Kussmaul: Deep and rapid; associated with metabolic acidosis
Cheyne-Stokes: Rhythmic waxing and waning from deep to shallow followed by a temporary period of apnea
Orthopnea: Requires upright position to breathe
Dyspnea: Difficulty breathing

Blood Pressure

Normal: Systolic blood pressure (SBP) <120 mm Hg; diastolic blood pressure (DBP) <80 mm Hg

Prehypertension: SBP 120–139 mm Hg or DBP 80–89 mm Hg

Stage 1 hypertension: SBP 140–159 mm Hg or DBP 90–99 mm Hg

Stage 2 hypertension: SBP ≥160 mm Hg or DBP ≥100 mm Hg

Pulse pressure: Difference between systolic and diastolic pressures

Fever

- ↑ temp; low-grade fever is 98.6°F–101°F; high-grade fever >101°F
- **Etiology:** Bacterial, viral, or fungal infection; deep vein thrombosis (DVT); medication side effects; tumor
- **S&S:** Fatigue; weakness; flushed, dry skin

Nursing Care

- Assess VS and WBCs; evaluate medications for possible drug-induced fever.
- Obtain diagnostic tests such as sputum, blood, or urine for culture and sensitivity (C&S), chest x-ray.
- Perform focused assessments: ↓ breath sounds; crackles; rhonchi; stiff neck; headache; photophobia; irritability; confusion; check IV site, incisions, and wounds for infection; check legs for DVT such as redness, warmth, swelling, tenderness; assess for urinary tract infection such as burning on urination, cloudy, greenish/reddish color; GI S&S such as diarrhea, N&V, abdominal discomfort.
- Institute seizure precautions for infants and toddlers if temperature is >101.8°F.
- Encourage coughing and deep breathing; ↑ fluid intake.
- Give prescribed antipyretics, antibiotics, tepid bath, hypothermia blanket.
- Change IV site if indicated.

Constipation

- ≤2 stools a week; difficult passage of hardened, dry stool; intractable constipation **(obstipation).**
- **Etiology:** Ignored urge; ↓ fluids or fiber in diet; ↓ mobility; weak abdominal or pelvic floor muscles; medication side effects such as opioids, iron, monoamine oxidase (MAO) inhibitors; anal lesions; pregnancy; laxative or enema abuse; F&E imbalance; intestinal obstruction.
  - **Infant and child:** Formula feeding; breastfed infants may have infrequent BMs due to digestibility of breast milk; stool-withholding behavior.

■ **S&S:** Hard/dry feces; distended abdomen; rectal pressure or fullness; back pain; straining at stool; anorexia; blood-streaked stools; ↓ bowel sounds.

Nursing Care

■ Assess stools for frequency, amount, color, consistency, shape.
■ Assess bowel and dietary habits such as preferred foods, formula vs. breast milk.
■ Teach to ↑ intake of fiber such as whole grain cereal, bran, vegetables, raw fruit, dried prunes; avoid binding foods such as rice, bananas; ↑ fluids; ↑ activity.
■ Teach to respond to urge; encourage sitting position and regular time (best in a.m. or after meal); ↑ relaxation and privacy.
■ Teach parents of infants that transient constipation resolves spontaneously and mild constipation resolves with introduction of solid foods; inform them that rectal stimulation with cotton-tipped applicator or thermometer is contraindicated because it can cause pain and anal fissures.
■ Give prescribed stool softeners, laxatives, cathartics, enemas.

Diarrhea

■ Passage of fluid or unformed stool >3 a day.
■ **Etiology**
   Acute (sudden onset): Viral, bacterial, or parasitic pathogen (usually spread via fecal-oral route or direct person-to-person contact); contaminated food or water; spicy, greasy food; raw seafood; excessive roughage; anxiety; medication side effects of antibiotics, laxatives, cathartics; environment (attends day care, recent travel).
   Chronic (persistent, recurrent): Malabsorption syndrome; food allergies such as lactose, gluten; inflammatory bowel disease such as ulcerative colitis, Crohn disease; AIDS.
■ **S&S:** Frequent, loose stool; foul-smelling, bulky stool indicates malabsorption; perianal excoriation; abdominal pain or cramps; flatus; abdominal distention; ↑ bowel sounds; N&V; anorexia; ↓ weight; fatigue and lethargy; ↑T; ↑ P; ↑ R; manifestations of dehydration.

Nursing Care

■ Assess stools for frequency, amount, color, consistency; VS; S&S of dehydration.
■ Provide oral rehydration therapy.
■ Assess perianal skin breakdown; provide skin care.
■ Ask about dietary intake and recent foreign travel; teach about ordered dietary restrictions such as lactose—milk and dairy products; gluten—wheat, rye, barley.

- Obtain stool specimen for C&S, ova and parasites; obtain specimen before giving prescribed antibiotic.
- Encourage breastfeeding mother to continue breastfeeding.
- Give prescribed antidiarrheals, antibiotics, IV fluids, electrolytes.
- Institute contact precautions as indicated.

Hemorrhage

- Bleeding that compromises tissue and organ perfusion.
- **Etiology**
  External: Surgical and traumatic wounds.
  Internal: Blunt trauma; cancer; ruptured aneurysm; GI perforation; thrombolytic therapy.
- **S&S:** ↑ P; ↑ R; ↓ BP; narrowing pulse pressure; excessive blood loss; capillary refill >3 seconds; ↓ peripheral pulses; cool, moist, pale, mottled, or cyanotic skin; thirst.
  Early CNS S&S: ↓ LOC; anxiety; irritability; restlessness.
  Late CNS S&S: Confusion; lethargy; combativeness; coma.

Nursing Care

- Apply direct pressure; reinforce dressing (removal may dislodge clot).
- Assess VS, I&O, lab results such as arterial blood gases, RBC, Hct, Hb, potassium.
- Maintain airway; give oxygen.
- Ensure 18-gauge IV access; give prescribed IVF, blood and blood products, colloidal products, vasoconstrictors, cardiac stimulants.

Shock

- Acute circulatory collapse; ↓ oxygen to cells, tissues, and organs.
- **Etiology**
  Hypovolemic: Blood loss; dehydration.
  Neurogenic: Spinal cord injury; anesthesia.
  Anaphylactic: Exposure to antigen.
  Septic: Infection; endo/exotoxin release.
  Cardiogenic: Heart fails as a pump.

- **S&S of all types:** ↓ BP, urinary output; capillary refill >3 seconds; cool, pale, mottled, or cyanotic skin; change in mental status.
  Hypovolemic: ↓ peripheral pulses.
  Neurogenic: Tachycardia or bradycardia.
  Anaphylactic: Anxiety; throat tightness; stridor; tachypnea; diaphoresis; flushing; urticaria; coma.

Septic: Fever; tachycardia; tachypnea.
Cardiogenic: Distended jugular and peripheral veins; pulmonary edema.

Nursing Care

■ **Emergency intervention**: Establish airway; suction if needed; give oxygen via nonrebreather mask 10–15 L/min; place in supine position with legs elevated unless airway compromised, then low Fowler; maintain IV access with 18-gauge needle; prepare for code, intubation, central venous access; give prescribed IVF and emergency medications; transfer to ICU.

■ **Ongoing assessments:** ECG; hemodynamic monitoring; LOC; orientation; VS; pulse oximetry (may be unreliable due to ↓ peripheral perfusion); I&O; skin for color, temperature, turgor, moistness.

■ **Specific to types:**
Hypovolemic: Control bleeding if present; give prescribed colloids, plasma expanders, and/or blood products.
Neurogenic: Spinal stabilization; give prescribed vasopressors.
Anaphylactic: Give prescribed epinephrine, antihistamines, steroids.
Septic: Give prescribed volume replacement, antibiotics, vasopressors, antipyretics.
Cardiogenic: Give prescribed vasopressors, cardiotonics, antidysrhythmics.

Infection

■ Entry and multiplication of a pathogen in tissue; can be local or systemic or progress from local to systemic such as UTIs can spread to kidneys and bloodstream; infection is accompanied by the inflammatory response.

■ **Etiology:** Invasion by bacterial, viral, or fungal pathogen.

■ **S&S**
Local: Erythema; edema; tenderness; heat; ↓ function; purulent exudate; positive culture; S&S also depend on tissue involved.
Systemic: ↑VS; chills; diaphoresis; malaise; ↑WBCs; positive culture; occasionally headache; muscle/joint pain; changes in mental status.

Nursing Care

■ Assess VS, S&S of inflammation and infection.
■ Obtain C&S before first dose of antibiotic if infection is suspected.
■ Avoid excess bedcovers; change linen if diaphoretic.
■ Promote rest and immobilization.
■ Give prescribed oxygen, IVF, ↑ oral fluids, ↑ protein, vitamin C, wound care.
■ Transmission-based precautions as indicated.

Inflammatory Response

- Local vascular response to protect and repair tissue; inflammatory response can occur with or without an infection.
- Progression of response:
  - Offending factor precipitates release of histamine, prostaglandin, bradykinin, and serotonin, which cause blood vessel dilation and ↑ vascular permeability.
  - Fluids, protein, and cells move from the intravascular compartment to interstitial tissue, causing local edema, heat, redness.
  - ↑ interstitial fluid and histamine put pressure on and irritate nerve endings, resulting in pain; pain and edema ↓ function.
  - Formation of inflammatory exudates such as pus and serum occurs.
- **Etiology:** Physical trauma, chemical agents, microorganisms.
- **S&S:** Local edema; heat; redness; pain; ↓ function; exudate may be clear, plasmalike **(serous)**; pink with RBCs **(serosanguineous)**; yellowish green with WBCs and bacteria **(purulent, pus)**; ↑ temperature and purulent exudate indicate infection.

Nursing Care

- Assess for S&S of inflammation and infection; wound characteristics.
- Provide ordered wound care.
- Elevate area if possible to ↓ edema; immobilize area to ↓ pain.
- Give prescribed antipyretics, anti-inflammatories, antibiotics.
- Perform prescribed thermal applications:
  Cold: At time of injury to ↑ vasoconstriction which ↓ pain and edema.
  Warm: After 24–48 hours to ↑ circulation which removes debris and localizes inflammatory agents.

Nausea and Vomiting

- Unpleasant wavelike sensation in throat and epigastrium **(nausea)**; ejection of GI contents through mouth **(vomiting, emesis)**; when ejected with force **(projectile vomiting)**; vomiting ↑ risk for aspiration resulting in atelectasis, pneumonia, asphyxiation; complications include dehydration, electrolyte imbalances, metabolic alkalosis.
- **Etiology:** Gastroenteritis; motion sickness; pain; stress; medication side effects; pregnancy; gastrointestinal obstructions such as pyloric stenosis, tumors, intussusception, volvulus; neurological causes such as increased intracranial pressure, head trauma, vascular headache; gastrointestinal diseases such as appendicitis, peptic ulcers.
- **S&S:** N&V; salivation; ↑↓ P; pallor; diaphoresis; hyperactive, high-pitched bowel sounds; abdominal pain; manifestations of F&E imbalance such as

hypokalemia, metabolic alkalosis; visible peristaltic waves with projectile vomiting.
■ **Color of vomitus:**
Red—frank bleeding.
Coffee grounds—blood acted on by gastric enzymes.
Green bilious—contains bile.

Nursing Care
■ Stay with patient; provide physical and emotional support.
■ Maintain airway; ↑ head of bed or place in side-lying position to prevent aspiration.
■ Assess emesis amount and characteristics; note if vomiting is projectile.
■ Keep NPO; assess hydration status, I&O, VS, electrolytes, daily weight.
■ Assess abdomen for distention, tenderness, intestinal peristalsis.
■ Assess in relation to food, medications, toxic substances.
■ Provide oral and physical hygiene; lubricate lips with water-soluble jelly.
■ Notify primary health-care provider; obtain prescription for alternate route for po medications.
■ Give prescribed IVF, antiemetic; reintroduce ordered fluids and foods slowly.

Deficit Fluid Volume (Dehydration)

■ ↓ Intravascular, interstitial, and/or intracellular fluid.
■ **Types:**
Isotonic: Fluid and electrolyte deficits in balanced proportions.
Hypotonic: Electrolyte deficit exceeds fluid deficit.
Hypertonic: Fluid loss exceeds electrolyte loss.
■ **Etiology:** ↓ fluid absorption; ↓ fluid intake; GI losses from vomiting; diarrhea; nasogastric tube suction; ↑ urine output due to diabetes mellitus and inappropriate ADH secretion; diaphoresis or excessive evaporative losses from fever, hyperventilation; ↑ environmental temperature; hemorrhage.
Infant: Use of radiant warmer or phototherapy.
■ **S&S:** Vary by degree of dehydration; dry mucous membranes; furrowed tongue; ↓ thirst (not reliable in older adult); rapid weight loss; muscle weakness; lethargy; flat neck veins in supine position; narrow pulse pressure; orthostatic hypotension; urinary output exceeds intake if this is the cause of the fluid volume deficit.

Assessment Factor	Mild Dehydration	Moderate Dehydration	Severe Dehydration
% of fluid loss	Infant: 5%–6% Child: 3%–4% Adult: 2%–3%	Infant: 10% Child: 6%–8% Adult: 5%–6%	Infant: ≥15% Child: ≥10% Adult: >8%
Fluid volume loss	<50 mL/kg	50–100 mL/kg	>100 mL/kg
Blanch test	<2 seconds	2–3 seconds	>3 seconds
Skin turgor has delayed return to normal after pinch (tenting)	**Estimate % of total body weight loss** (not accurate in older adults) <2 seconds: <5% 2–3 seconds: 5%–8% 3–4 seconds: 9%–10% >4 seconds: >10%		
Skin color	Normal	Pale	Gray, mottled
Fontanels (infants)	Normal or depressed	Depressed	Depressed
Eyeballs	Normal or soft	Soft, sunken	Soft, sunken
Blood pressure	Normal	Normal or decreased	Decreased
Pulse	Normal or ↑ rate, strong strength	↑ rate, weak strength	↑ rate, easily obliterated on palpation (thready)
Respirations	Normal or ↑ rate	↑ rate	↑ rate
Urine output	Slightly ↓	Mild oliguria	Marked oliguria, anuria

Nursing Care

- Assess for S&S; determine degree of dehydration.
  Child or adult: 2 lb = 1 L of fluid.
  Infant: 1 g wet diaper weight = 1 mL urine.
- Monitor intake and output.
- Assess VS every 15–30 min until stable and then routine.
- Weigh routinely.
  Infant or child: Every 2 hours.
  Adult: Daily.
- Give prescribed oral replacement therapy (ORT).
  Infant or child: 50–100 mL/kg for mild to moderate dehydration.
  Adults: Encourage twice usual daily intake (at least 3000 mL).

- Give prescribed IV fluid replacement for severe dehydration.
  Infant or child: 1–3 boluses of NS or lactated Ringer, 20–30 mL/kg.
  Adult: Normal saline or Ringer solutions.
- Give prescribed sodium bicarbonate to correct metabolic acidosis; potassium replacement once kidney function and adequate circulation are ensured; rapid fluid replacement is contraindicated with hypertonic dehydration because of risk of water intoxication.
- Assess for S&S of water intoxication: ↑ urine output, irritability, somnolence, headache, vomiting, seizures.

Orthostatic Hypotension (Postural Hypotension)

- ↓ BP when rising from lying down to sitting or sitting to standing due to peripheral vasodilation without a compensatory ↑ cardiac output.
- **Etiology:** Older age; immobility; hypovolemia; anemia; dysrhythmias; medication side effect (opioids, antihypertensives, diuretics).
- **S&S:** light-headedness; vertigo; weakness; cool, pale, diaphoretic skin.

Nursing Care
- Assess for ↑ P and ↓ BP when changing position.
- Teach patient to rise slowly, sit for 1 min before standing, resume prior position if dizzy.
- Assist to bed, chair, or floor if falling; if ↓ BP continues, assess for ↓ LOC, neurological status, cardiac status, S&S of dehydration; notify primary health-care provider.

Prenatal Period: Fertilization to Start of Labor

Signs of Pregnancy

- **Presumptive signs:** Absence of menses **(amenorrhea)**; first awareness of fetal movement **(quickening)** by 16–20 weeks.
- **Probable signs:** Softening of cervix **(Goodell sign)**; bluish purple mucous membranes of cervix, vagina, vulva **(Chadwick sign)**; softening of lower-uterine segment **(Hegar sign)**; floating fetus rebounds against examiner's fingers **(ballottement)**.
- **Positive signs:** Fetal heart sounds; fetal movement; ultrasound of fetus.

Prenatal Physiological Progression

- Ovum expelled from graafian follicle (ovulation); then sperm unites with ovum (fertilization) in fallopian tube within 24 hr.
- Fertilized ovum attaches to uterine endometrium (implantation).
- Conceptus called embryo (first 8 weeks), then fetus.
- **Trimesters:** First (0–15 weeks); second (16–27 weeks); third (28–37/40 weeks).
- **Nägele Rule:** Expected date of birth (EDB); add 7 days to first day of last menstruation, subtract 3 months, add 1 yr.
- Cells differentiate weeks 3–8 (organogenesis); negative influences such as drugs and illness may cause defects in embryo (teratogens).
- Fetal heart audible with Doptone after 12 weeks.
- Fetal lungs produce pulmonary surfactants at 24–28 weeks.
- Deposits of brown fat begins at 28 weeks; most weight gain in third trimester.

Signs and Symptoms of Impending Labor

- Fetal presenting part descends into true pelvis (lightening).
- Cervix thins and shortens (effacement); external os opens (dilation).
- Mild, irregular uterine contractions (preparatory contractions), formerly Braxton Hicks.
- Energy spurt (nesting), usually 24–48 hr before labor.
- Expulsion of mucous plug, usually 24–48 hr before labor.

Prenatal Maternal Changes

Endocrine

- Placenta secretes human chorionic gonadotropin (hCG); used for pregnancy screening; has role in a.m. nausea.
- Progesterone and estrogen from corpus luteum in first trimester; from placenta in second and third trimesters.
- Thyroid, parathyroids, pancreas ↑ secretions; need for ↑ insulin.
- Estro levels ↑; excess in maternal saliva may indicate preterm labor.
- Labor initiated by posterior pituitary oxytocin; ↑ progesterone; ↑ estrogen; ↓ prostaglandins.

Nursing Care

- Obtain specimens for screening tests.

Circulatory

- Cardiac output ↑ 30%–50%; blood volume ↑ 50% and RBCS ↑ 30% (physiological anemia); ↓ hematocrit (Hct) level; white blood cells ↑ to 12,000 mm3.

- Palpitations in first trimester are due to SNS stimulation; in third trimester are due to ↑ thoracic pressure.
- Heart rate (HR) ↑ 10–15 bpm; BP decreases in latter half of pregnancy; HR may ↑ 40% with multiple fetuses.
- Supine hypotension syndrome **(vena cava syndrome)**: weight of uterus on vena cava ↓ venous return to heart and ↓ placental blood flow; S&S include ↓ BP, light-headedness, palpitations.
- Fibrinogen and other clotting factors ↑.
- Varicose veins of legs, vulva, perianal area **(hemorrhoids)** due to pressure of uterus on pelvic blood vessels.
- Edema of extremities last 6 weeks due to circulatory stasis.

Nursing Care
- Teach patient to ↑ fluids, change positions slowly, elevate legs, wear antiembolism stockings, avoid prolonged sitting and crossing legs; give prescribed anticoagulant.
- For deep venous thrombosis (DVT): Maintain bedrest, give prescribed anticoagulant.

Respiratory
- Oxygen consumption ↑ 15% by 16–40 weeks.
- Nasal congestion and epistaxis due to ↑ estrogen levels.
- Dyspnea due to enlarged uterus pressing against diaphragm; subsides when lightening occurs around 38 weeks.

Nursing Care
- Teach to balance rest and activity; avoid large meals.
- Suggest to blow nose gently; use saline nasal spray.

Reproductive
- Amenorrhea; leukorrhea.
- ↑ vaginal acidity protects against bacterial invasion.
- Cervical and uterine changes: Goodell, Chadwick, Hegar signs.
- Uterus in pelvic cavity at 12–14 weeks; then in abdominal cavity to umbilicus at 22–24 weeks and almost xiphoid process at term.
- Breast changes: Fullness; tingling; soreness; darkening of areolae and nipples; nipples more erect; veins more prominent; reddish stretch marks; Montgomery follicles enlarge.

Nursing Care
- Assess fundal height.
- Suggest side-lying, vaginal rear entry for intercourse.
- Teach not to douche; use a supportive brassiere and cotton underpants.

Gastrointestinal

- Nausea without vomiting (**morning sickness**) and ↓ salivation due to hormonal changes.
- Food cravings; eating substances not normally edible (**pica**).
- Heartburn and gastric reflux due to delayed emptying of stomach and pressure of uterus.
- Flatulence due to ↓ GI motility, air swallowing.
- Constipation due to ↑ peristalsis, pressure of uterus, hemorrhoids.

Nursing Care

- Teach to avoid gastric irritants, gas-forming foods, antacids containing sodium.
- Remain upright 1 hr after meals; small, frequent meals; dry crackers before arising if nauseated; ↑ fiber, fluid, walking to prevent constipation.
- For hemorrhoids: Avoid straining at stool and prolonged sitting; use warm sitz baths or ice packs; anesthetic ointments as prescribed.

Urinary

- Urinary frequency in early and late pregnancy due to enlarging uterus.
- Bladder capacity ↑ to 1500 mL due to ↑ bladder tone; may lead to stasis and infection.
- ↓ renal threshold may cause glycosuria and mild proteinuria.

Nursing Care

- Teach to void every 2 hr and on urge to prevent stasis.
- Assess for glycosuria due to diabetes and proteinuria due to preeclampsia.

Integumentary

- Blotchy, brownish skin over cheeks, nose, and forehead (**melasma, chloasma**); pigmented line from symphysis pubis to top of fundus in midline (**linea nigra**).
- Stretch marks over abdomen, thighs, breasts (**striae gravidarum**) due to adrenocorticosteroids during second half of pregnancy.
- ↑ perspiration; oily skin; hirsutism; acne vulgaris.

Nursing Care

- Teach that integumentary changes are common.
- Changes generally subside after birth; striae lighten.

Musculoskeletal

- Softening of all ligaments and joints, particularly symphysis pubis and sacroiliac joints; backache due to lordosis and changes in center of gravity; leg cramps due to hypocalcemia and pressure of uterus on pelvic nerves.

Nursing Care
- Encourage intake of calcium-rich foods and perinatal vitamin.
- Teach body mechanics, avoid high-heeled shoes and lifting.

Nutritional Needs
- 25–35 lb gain: 2–5 lb/week in first trimester; 3/4 lb/week in second to third trimesters.
- **Calories:** ↑ 300 calories daily to total of 2500 calories daily.
- **Protein:** 60 g daily, an increase of 14 g daily above pre-pregnant level.
- **Carbohydrates (CHO):** Adequate to meet requirements; complex CHO preferred.
- **Fats:** 30% of daily caloric intake; 10% should be saturated.
- **RDA vitamins and minerals:** Attained in balanced diet and perinatal vitamin containing 400 mcg folic acid; sodium is never completely restricted; avoid excess.

Nursing Care
- Teach patient to have well-balanced diet, avoid dieting.
- Teach patient to take multivitamin containing 400 mcg folic acid daily before conception and during pregnancy to prevent fetal neural tube defects.

Prenatal Health Promotion

- **Travel:** Lap belt under abdomen and shoulder belt between breasts; stand and walk briefly every hr; airlines may restrict travel close to EDB.
- **Smoking:** Avoid to prevent spontaneous abortion, ↓ birth weight, apnea in newborn.
- **Employment:** Avoid excessive standing or work that causes severe physical strain or fatigue.
- **Alcohol:** Avoid to prevent preterm birth; ↓ birth weight; fetal alcohol effect (FAE); fetal alcohol syndrome (FAS).
- **Illicit drugs:** Avoid to prevent teratogenic effect; ↓ birth weight; small for gestational age (SGA); fetal addiction or dependency.
- **Caffeine:** ↑ risk of spontaneous abortion and intrauterine growth restriction; FDA recommends ≤ 2–3 servings (200–300 mg) daily.
- **Artificial sweeteners:** Studies are inconclusive but moderation is recommended; mothers with phenylketonuria (PKU) should avoid aspartame.

Tests Performed During Pregnancy

Human Chorionic Gonadotropin (hCG, HCG)
- Tests for pregnancy; detectable 8 days after conception.
- Produced by cells covering the chorionic villi of placenta.
- Slowly elevating or ↓ levels: threatened abortion, ectopic pregnancy.
- ↑ levels: May indicate ectopic pregnancy; hydatidiform mole; Down syndrome.

Maternal Serum Alpha-Fetoprotein (AFP) Screening
- Fetal protein used to screen for neural tube defects.
- Ranges identified for each week of gestation.
- Peak concentrations at end of first trimester.
- 16–18 weeks optimum time for testing.
- ↑ levels: Risk of open neural tube defect.
- ↓ levels: Risk of Down syndrome; when ↓ levels persist, ultrasonography for structural anomalies and amniocentesis for chromosomal analysis are done.

Chorionic Villus Sampling
- Reflects fetal chromosomes; DNA; enzymology.
- Placental tissue aspirated at 10–12 weeks.
- Earlier testing time than amniocentesis permits earlier decision regarding termination.
- Also ↓ risk of first-trimester spontaneous abortion; costs less than amniocentesis.
- Complications: Infection; preterm labor.

Nursing Care
- Obtain consent.
- Encourage full bladder to serve as acoustic window.
- Assess vital signs; absence of uterine cramping.
- Provide emotional support; ensure genetic counseling if appropriate.
- Teach that spotting of blood for 3 days is expected after transcervical route; report flulike symptoms and vaginal discharge of blood, clots, tissue, or amniotic fluid; avoid sexual activity, lifting, or strenuous activity until spotting resolves.

Biophysical Profile (BPP)
- Indicted when there are S&S of fetal compromise.
- Ultrasonography assesses fetal breathing movements and tone, amniotic fluid volume, and gross body movement.
- Non-stress test assesses fetal heart rate reactivity.

- Fetus status reflected numerically like Apgar score.
- Reflects central nervous system integrity; indicator of fetal crisis or demise.

Nursing Care
- Same as fetal ultrasonography; provide emotional support.

Percutaneous Umbilical Blood Samplings (PUBS)
- Fetal cord blood assessed at >17 weeks; identifies some maternal and fetal problems.
- Complications: Bleeding, infection, thrombosis, preterm labor.

Nursing Care
- Obtain consent; full bladder may be necessary; assess uterine activity, fetal heart rate (FHR) and FHR reactivity.
- Teach to take antibiotics, temperature two times daily, report ↑ temperature.

Fetal Ultrasonography
- Serial exams document progress, gestational age, placenta location, fetal position, presentation.
- Assesses FHR, breathing movements, amniotic fluid index (AFI); estimates birth weight; visualizes multiple fetuses, maternal pelvic masses, gross fetal structural parts and abnormalities; pockets of amniotic fluid; fetal demise.

Nursing Care
- Education based on findings; provide emotional support.
- Transabdominal: Drink 1–2 L fluid 1 hr before test to fill bladder.
- Transvaginal: Empty bladder to ↑ view of uterus.
- Place a wedge underneath maternal hip if in third trimester to decrease compression of the vena cava.

Amniocentesis
- Analysis of amniotic fluid.
- **14–17 weeks:** Identifies chromosomal and biochemical disorders such as Down syndrome and neural tube defects, fetal age, gender, ↑ bilirubin such as Rh disease, and intra-amniotic infections.
- **≥35 weeks:** Lecithin/sphingomyelin (L/S) ratio of 2:1, phosphatidyl glycerol (PG) present, and lamellar bodies of over 35,000 particles/mcL; all indicate lung maturity.
- Complications: preterm labor, amniotic fluid emboli, infection.

Nursing Care
- Obtain consent.
- **14–17 weeks:** Bladder must be full to raise uterus toward abdominal cavity. Second half of pregnancy:
  - Tell patient to empty bladder to ↓ confusion with uterus; hip roll to ↓ hypotension.

- Assess maternal VS, fetal cardiac activity.
- Teach that mild cramping is common; fluid leakage usually is self-limiting.
- Tell patient to avoid intercourse, heavy lifting, strenuous activity for 24 hr after test; report ↑ temperature, persistent cramping, or vaginal discharge.
- Ensure genetic counseling if appropriate; provide emotional support.

Amniotic Fluid Tests
- **Nitrazine test:** Positive test tape dark blue or gray/green.
- **Fern test:** Fern pattern under microscope.

Nursing Care
- Dorsal lithotomy position; encourage coughing to ↑ fluid expulsion.
- Touch nitrazine tape to vaginal secretions; for fern test, use cotton-tipped applicator to collect secretions and draw over glass slide.

Fetal Fibronectin (fFN)
- Swab of vaginal and cervical secretions done at 22–31 weeks; fFN leaks with amniotic sac separation; presence may predict labor onset.

Nursing Care
- Assist with dorsal recumbent or lithotomy position.
- Collect sample like a Pap smear.

Nonstress Test (NST)
- Done after 28 weeks; Doppler transducer records FHR in relation to movement; tocotransducer records fetal movement as changes in uterine pressure.
- Test results:
  - **Reactive NST:** Two accelerations (↑ of 15 bpm for 15 seconds) in 20 min and normal baseline FHR; predictive of fetal well-being.
  - **Nonreactive NST:** Failure to meet reactive criteria over 40 min; vibro-acoustic stimulus for 1 second may be used to startle fetus, which can be repeated two times.
  - **Inconclusive:** <2 accelerations in 20 min; accelerations do not meet reactive criteria; inadequate quality recording for interpretation.

Nursing Care
- Left lateral position to ↓ vena cava compression; transducer and tocody-namometer to abdomen; teach to press event button with fetal movement.

Contraction Stress Test (CST)
- Contractions stimulated and fetal response monitored; done after nonreactive NST; identifies if fetus can withstand ↓ oxygen during stress of contraction.
- Test results:
  - **Negative:** Normal baseline FHR, FHR accelerations with fetal movement, and no late decelerations with three contractions in 10 min indicates

healthy fetus; oxytocin discontinued; IV continued until uterine activity returns to prior status; fetus likely to survive labor if it occurs within 1 week with no maternal or fetal change.

- ■ **Positive**: Late decelerations with 50% of contractions indicate a nonreassuring fetal sign; assess mother and fetus; prepare for labor induction.
- ■ **Suspicious**: Late decelerations with less than half the contractions.

Nursing Care
- ■ Obtain consent; semi-Fowler position with lateral tilt; Doppler transducer to abdomen; baseline and every 30 min maternal VS and FHR.
- ■ Assist with stimulation; assess IV and mother for S&S of preterm labor.

Fetal Movement Count
- ■ 28 weeks fetal movement counted by patient at same time daily; more testing indicated for ≤ three fetal movements.

Nursing Care
- ■ Teach patient to assume a comfortable position; hands on abdomen; count number of fetal movements in 1 hr.

Doppler Studies (Umbilical Vessel Velocimetry)
- ■ Measures blood flow velocity and direction in uterine and fetal structures.
- ■ ↓ umbilical vessel flow seen in intrauterine growth restriction (IUGR), preeclampsia, eclampsia, post-term.

Nursing Care
- ■ Same as fetal ultrasonography.

Potential Problems During Pregnancy

Disseminated Intravascular Coagulation (DIC)
- ■ ↑ clotting in microcirculation; platelets and clotting factors become depleted → bleeding and thromboemboli in organs; ↑ risk for DIC in abruptio placentae.
- ■ **S&S**: Bleeding, petechiae, ecchymosis, purpura, occult blood, hematuria, hematemesis, shock, ↑ PT, ↑ PTT, ↓ platelet count, ↓ hematocrit and ↓ fibrinogen levels.

Nursing Care
- ■ Assess for S&S, VS changes, shock.
- ■ Give oxygen and prescribed medications.

Fetal Demise: Fetal Death in Utero (FDIU)
- ■ Birth of dead fetus >20 weeks gestation or weight ≤350 g **(stillbirth)**.
- ■ **S&S**: No fetal movement or FHR; ↓ fundal height; ↓ fetal growth; may spontaneously go into labor within 2 weeks or may be induced.

Nursing Care
- Assess for S&S.
- Encourage expression of feelings; support grieving and memories such as seeing, holding, naming, memory box (pictures, blanket, clothing, ID bands, hair lock).
- Provide for privacy; ensure that family needs are met; refer to support group.

Hyperemesis Gravidarum
- Intractable N&V beyond first trimester causing F&E and nutritional imbalance.
- **S&S:** N&V; ↓ weight; fluid volume deficit (FVD); electrolyte and acid-base imbalances; ↑ Hct; ketonuria.

Nursing Care
- Assess for S&S.
- NPO until dehydration resolves and 48 hr after vomiting stops; encourage dry diet if tolerated; advance to small amounts of alternating fluids and solids.
- Give ordered IV fluid replacement and prescribed antiemetics.

Multiple Gestation
- Multiple fetuses due to multiple ovulation, splitting of fertilized egg(s), or multiple in vitro implantations.
- **S&S:** Excessive fetal activity and uterine size; ↑ weight; multiple FHRs; palpation of 3–4 large fetal parts in uterus.

Nursing Care
- Assess VS, fetal growth, S&S of preterm labor, nonreassuring fetal signs.
- Prepare for cesarean birth; give prescribed oxytocic meds postpartum to prevent hemorrhage because of atony due to excessive uterine distention.

Trophoblastic Disease
- Abnormal growth of tissue and ↑ βhCG; hydatidiform mole.
- Risk factors include ovulation stimulation, early teens, or ≥40 yr of age.
- **S&S:** Uterus large for gestational age; no FHR, movement, or palpable parts; hypertension (HTN); hyperemesis; vaginal passage of grapelike substance common; confirmed by ultrasonography.
- ↑ risk for hemorrhage; perforation; infection; choriocarcinoma.

Nursing Care
- Assist with suction curettage; avoid induction due to risk of embolization.
- Measurement of βhCG for 1 yr after expulsion; encourage to avoid pregnancy for 1 yr to allow assessments for S&S of choriocarcinoma.

Ectopic Pregnancy

- Implantation outside uterus; mid-fallopian tube most common site.
- **S&S:** Early signs may be obscure; spotting after 1–2 missed periods; sudden, knifelike right or left lower abdominal pain radiating to shoulder (tube rupture); rigid abdomen; shock with obscured hemorrhage.

Nursing Care

- Assess for S&S, VS for shock, pain pattern, anxiety.
- Give prescribed transfusions, pain medications, RhoGAM to Rh-negative patient if appropriate; prepare for repair or removal of tube.

Infections That Are Teratogenic

Toxoplasmosis

Protozoal infection; can cause spontaneous abortion in early pregnancy; transmitted via feces of infected cats and raw meat.

Nursing Care

- Avoid cat litter; cook meat well.

Rubella

Viral infection; teratogenic in first trimester; congenital defects in heart, ears, eyes, brain.

Nursing Care

- Vaccination ≥3 months before pregnancy or after giving birth.
- Avoid people with rubella.

Cytomegalovirus (CMV)

Viral infection acquired via respiratory or sexual route; fetus may contract infection through birth canal; can cause retardation, deafness, heart defects, death of neonate.

Nursing Care

- Teach to avoid others with flulike infections.

Genital Herpes

Viral infection causing painful, draining vesicles on external genitalia, vagina, cervix; fetal-neonatal risk is greater when first outbreak occurs during pregnancy; fatal or permanent CNS damage if neonate is infected during vaginal birth.

Nursing Care

- During active infection: Use contact precautions, prepare for cesarean birth, separate mother with active lesions from neonate after birth.

Human Immunodeficiency Virus (HIV)

Viral infection; ↑ transmission risk with high viral load and prolonged ruptured membranes; antiviral therapy in second to third trimesters and neonate treatment for 6 weeks postbirth ↓ transmission by 66%.

Nursing Care

- ■ Encourage prenatal care, taking of all medications to ↓ viral load, health promotion to ↓ opportunistic infections.
- ■ Referrals for HIV counseling especially if acquired via risky behavior.

Vena Cava Syndrome (Supine Hypotensive Syndrome)

- ■ Partial occlusion of vena cava from pressure of uterus.
- ■ **S&S:** ↑ P; ↓ BP; N&V; diaphoresis; respiratory distress; nonreassuring fetal signs.

Nursing Care

- ■ Position on left side to shift weight of fetus off inferior vena cava.
- ■ Assess VS, FHR, S&S of shock; give oxygen.

Hypertensive Disorders (Includes Preeclampsia and Eclampsia)

- ■ Maternal BP ≥140/90 mm Hg.
- ■ Risk factors: Primipara <17 yr, >35 yr, multipara, DM, chronic HTN, multiple fetuses, trophoblastic or kidney disease, inadequate nutrition, Rh incompatibility.
- ■ Onset 12–24 weeks; subsides 6th week postpartum; only cure is birth of neonate.

Preeclampsia

- ■ S&S for mild: 140/90 mm Hg or higher; 1+ proteinuria; upper-body edema; progressive excessive weight gain.
- ■ S&S for severe: Two resting BP readings 6 hr apart ≥ 160/110 mm Hg; 3–4+ proteinuria; massive generalized edema; oliguria; sudden large weight gain; CNS irritability such as headache, blurred vision, hyperreflexia.

Eclampsia

- ■ Seizure in pregnancy not attributable to another cause.
- ■ **HELLP syndrome: H**emolysis of RBCs, **E**levated **L**iver enzymes, **L**ow **P**latelets; variant of severe preeclampsia; multiorgan failure.

Nursing Care for Patients With a Hypertensive Disorder

- ■ Assess VS and BP every 15 min when critical, then every 1–4 hr; assess edema (I&O, daily weight); CNS irritability such as vision problems and hyperreflexia; proteinuria; fetal status; hematological studies; signs of bleeding or labor.
- ■ Institute seizure precautions; provide quiet environment; limit visitors.
- ■ Encourage ↑ protein and moderate sodium intake; give prescribed magnesium sulfate ($MgSO_4$); give ordered oxygen.

- Assess for magnesium sulfate (MgSO$_4$) toxicity: Depressed or absent deep tendon reflexes; R <12 bpm; drug blood level >8 mg/dL (therapeutic range 48 mg/dL); keep calcium gluconate available as antidote for MgSO$_4$.
- Maintain bedrest in side-lying position during labor and birth; be prepared for cesarean birth; assess for 48 hr postpartum.
- Provide emotional support.

Incompetent Cervix
- Premature dilation-effacement of cervix; cervix may be sutured closed (**cerclage**) usually at 10–14 weeks gestation; sutures are removed at 37 weeks.
- **S&S:** Painless contractions; vaginal bleeding 18–28 weeks; fetal membranes observed through cervix.

Nursing Care
- Assess for S&S, nonreassuring fetal signs; maintain bedrest; prepare for suturing of cervix.
- Postop cerclage: Maintain bedrest for 24 hr; assess for ruptured membranes, contractions, vaginal bleeding; teach to avoid intercourse, lifting, prolonged standing as ordered.

Termination (Abortion and Assisted Abortion)
- Spontaneous or planned expulsion of products of conception.
- Treatment: Mifepristone (RU 486) first 9 weeks; minisuction first 5–7 weeks; vacuum aspiration first 12 weeks; dilation and curettage (D&C) 12–14 weeks; saline injection 14–24 weeks.

Nursing Care
- Assess VS, S&S of bleeding and infection, expelled products, pain, F&E balance.
- Give prescribed RhoGAM to Rh-negative mother; support grieving.

Labor and Birth

Stages of Labor

Nursing Care Common to All Stages
- Establish trust; answer questions; support mother and coach; inform parents and primary health-care provider of progress.
- Use standard precautions.
- Assess contractions; dilation; engagement; position and presentation; fetal and maternal VS (assess between contractions, normal FHR 120–160 bpm); S&S of dehydration, edema.

- Provide fluids per orders; encourage voiding every 1–2 hr.
- For ↓ BP: Turn on side and retake.
- For pulse oximetry <90% provide oxygen.
- For ruptured membranes: Assess for prolapsed cord; meconium-stained amniotic fluid (a nonreassuring fetal sign); S&S of infection; fetal monitoring: See Fetal Heart Rate (FHR) Monitoring, p. 62.

Stage 1: Begins With Regular Contractions and Ends With Fully Dilated Cervix

Phase and Description	Nursing Care
Latent phase: Mild to moderate contractions; every 15–30 min, 15–30 sec long; dilation 0–3 cm. **Mother:** Alert; excited; verbalizes concerns; may rest or sleep; uses relaxation techniques.	• Encourage ambulation and upright position if no ruptured membranes. • Review breathing and focusing techniques. • Offer ordered fluids and food. • Assess fetal presentation and position **(Leopold maneuvers).**
Active phase: Moderate to strong contractions; every 3–5 min, up to 60 sec long; dilation 4–7 cm; membranes may rupture. **Mother:** Alert; more demanding; anxious; restless; may seek pain relief; uses breathing and focusing techniques.	• Assist with position changes, hygiene, oral care. Provide ordered fluids. • Provide counterpressure to sacrococcygeal area, pillow support, and backrubs. • Offer and explain prescribed pain meds. • Talk through contractions. • Initiate hydrotherapy if desired. • Encourage breathing and focusing techniques.
Transition phase: Strong contractions; every 1–2 min; 45–60 sec long; dilation 8–10 cm. **Mother:** Restless; agitated; may have sudden N&V and pressure on rectum; has difficulty following directions and focusing.	• Stay with patient; accept irritability. • Use relaxation techniques such as effleurage between contractions. • Teach to pant to avoid premature pushing. • Provide supportive care for N&V and pain relief as indicated. • Prepare for birth.

Stage 2: Begins When Cervix Is Fully Dilated and Effaced and Ends With Birth of Fetus (Pushing Stage)

Description	Nursing Care
Dilation complete; progress determined by descent through birth canal **(fetal station)**; strong contractions every 2–3 min, 60–75 sec long; ↑ bloody show; fetal head visible **(crowning)**. **Mother:** Relaxes between but pushes with contractions; may report severe pain or burning sensation as perineum distends.	• Perform assessments every 5 min; assess FHR before, during, and after contractions. • Note duration, intensity, frequency of contractions with continuous monitoring device. • Assist to position that aids pushing. • Assess for crowning; encourage panting during contraction because it avoids precipitous birth; bearing down with contractions promotes birth. • Prepare for birth; offer mirror to see birth.

Stage 3: Begins at Birth of Neonate and Ends With Delivery of Placenta (Placental Stage)

Description	Nursing Care
Contractions every 3–4 min. Placental separation and expulsion: Firming and upward movement of fundus; rush of blood from vagina; lengthening umbilical cord; ↓ bleeding as uterus shrinks. May have perineal laceration or prophylactic incision **(episiotomy)**.	• Assess neonate (see Apgar, p. 75 and • Assessment of the Newborn, p. 76). • Assess mother: VS, fundal tone, contractions until placental delivery. • Assist to bear down to deliver placenta. • Give prescribed oxytocic and analgesic. • Keep mother and neonate warm. • Promote bonding before eye prophylaxis. • Put to breast if desired (skin-to-skin). • Assess parental reaction.

Stage 4: First 4 Hr After Placental Delivery (Recovery Stage)

Description	Nursing Care
↑ BP and slight tachycardia expected. Fundus midline, halfway between umbilicus and symphysis pubis; fundus should remain firm and contracted. **Red lochia (lochia rubra)** scant to moderate amount. Expected blood loss 250–500 mL.	• VS q 15 min for 1 hr. • **Fundus:** Should be 2 fingerbreadths below umbilicus. • **Bleeding:** <2 pads/hr, no free-flow or clots with fundal massage. • **Perineum:** Sutures intact, no bulging, slight bruising. • **Bladder:** Spontaneous voiding >100 mL; nondistended; uterus above umbilicus and to the right of midline indicates a full bladder; encourage voiding or catheterize if ordered. • **Discomfort:** tolerable, <3 on 0–10 pain scale; generally no severe pain. • Provide hygiene.

Fetal Heart Rate

Fetal Heart Rate (FHR) Monitoring
- **FHR monitoring:** Number of fetal heartbeats per minute; reflects fetal status and, indirectly, a supportive or nonsupportive uterine environment.
- **Auscultation:** Obtained by Doppler at 8–12 weeks; obtained by fetoscope at 16–20 weeks.
- **Intrapartum electronic monitoring:** Patterns reflect expected and abnormal fetal responses during labor; frequency and duration of contractions; FHR variability.
- **External monitor:** Ultrasound transducer on abdomen over fetal heart; tocotransducer over uterine fundus.
- **Internal monitor:** Electrode attached to fetal scalp after rupture of membranes.

FHR Patterns
- **Baseline FHR:** FHR between contractions.
- **Normal FHR:** 120–160 bpm; can be ↑ for short periods <10 min.

- **Tachycardia:** Sustained FHR >160 for >10 min; etiologies: early fetal hypoxia, immaturity, amnionitis, maternal fever, terbutaline sulfate.
- **Bradycardia:** Sustained FHR <120 for >10 min; etiologies: late or profound fetal hypoxia, maternal hypotension, prolonged cord compression, drugs, anesthetics.
- **Accelerations:** ↑ FHR 15 bpm and duration of 15 seconds; begins with contraction onset and returns to baseline at end of contraction; this is an expected fetal response.
- **Decelerations:** ↓ FHR in response to onset, peak, or relaxation of contractions or fetal activity.
- **Early onset:** Fetal head compression; generally benign. **Second stage:** If close together, stop patient from pushing until FHR returns to normal; rule out cephalopelvic disproportion if head is above ischial spines.
- **Variable:** Rapid onset and rapid return with variable relationship to contraction; OK if FHR baseline is acceptable; if it lasts >30 seconds or recovery to baseline is slow, notify primary health-care provider because it may indicate cord compromise such as cord prolapse, around fetal neck or shoulder, knotted. **If due to cord compression:** Stop oxytocin; lateral position; provide oxygen and IV fluids; prepare for cesarean birth if not corrected.
- **Late onset:** Starts at height of contraction and returns to baseline after contraction ends; reflects uteroplacental insufficiency.

Interventions Associated With Labor

Labor Induction
- Ripen cervix: Vaginal insertion of E1: misoprostol (Cytotec); or E2: dinoprostone (Prepidil, Cervidil).
- ↑ contractions once uterus is inducible: Amniotomy; oxytocin (Pitocin).
- Indications: Post-term, preeclampsia, eclampsia, intrauterine growth restriction, DM, fetal demise.
- Contraindications: Placenta previa, prolapsed cord, transverse fetal lie, active genital herpes, vertical cesarean scar.
- Complications: Contractions <2 min apart or lasting >90 seconds **(uterine tetany);** nausea; ↓ urine output.

Nursing Care
- Assess fetal and maternal response; discontinue oxytocin with uterine tetany.
- Place in left side-lying position; give oxygen; prepare for cesarean birth.

Augmentation of Labor
- Accelerate labor once it has begun; give prescribed oxytocin.
- Indications: Prolonged or dysfunctional labor, failure to dilate.
- Contraindications, complications, and nursing care same as labor induction.

Artificial Rupture of Membranes (AROM, Amniotomy)
- Indications: Hasten labor; permit internal fetal monitoring.
- Complication: Risk for infection the longer it takes to give birth.

Nursing Care
- Assess for cord prolapse and FHR.
- Maintain horizontal position; provide perineal care.

Forceps and Vacuum-Assisted Birth
- Forceps: Instruments are used to encircle fetal head; gentle pulling on handles helps extract neonate from birth canal.
- Vacuum: Soft cup applied over posterior fontanelle; gentle traction applied during maternal pushing; discontinued after three pulls, 20 min, three cup detachments or observed scalp trauma; helps extract neonate from birth canal.
- Maternal indications: Prolonged second stage, fatigue, maternal illness.
- Fetal indications: Nonreassuring FHR.
- Complications: Vaginal and rectal lacerations, fetal injury.

Nursing Care
- Assess for S&S of complications.
- Provide emotional support.
- Forceps: Assess FHR to ensure cord is not compressed.
- Vacuum: Teach mother that chignon will resolve in 3–7 days.

Cesarean Birth
- Birth via abdominal incision; low transverse incision most common; vertical incision ↑ risk of uterine rupture in future pregnancies.
- Indications: Stalled labor progress **(dystocia),** repeat cesarean birth, breech presentation, fetal compromise, active genital herpes, placenta previa, abruptio placentae, cord prolapse, preeclampsia, eclampsia.
- Complications: Wound infection, dehiscence, hemorrhage, bladder or bowel injury, thrombophlebitis, pulmonary embolus, fetal injury or aspiration.

Nursing Care
- Emphasis on healthy neonate and mother; assess for S&S of complications.
- Teach about surgery, anesthesia, recovery.

Labor and Birth: Analgesia and Anesthesia

Additional obstetrical medications presented in Tab 7, MEDS, Obstetric Medication, p. 272.

Epidural Block/Infusion

Injection of anesthetic into epidural space to ↓ pain of labor and birth.

Advantages: Titratable level; patient is awake; nausea and sedation are minimal; urge to push may be preserved; no headache.

Disadvantages: Maternal ↓ BP; labor progress and fetal descent may be slowed; less effective pushing in second stage; may cause N&V, pruritus, urinary retention.

Nursing Care

- Have patient void before; assess for bladder distention routinely.
- Minimize hypotension by giving 500–1000 mL IV fluids 15–30 min before placement as ordered; maintain side-lying position; alternate sides.
- Assist to side-lying or sitting position and support during insertion (patient must remain still); time insertion between contractions.
- Use an infusion pump; ensure catheter placement remains intact.
- Assess VS before, every 1–2 min for first 10 min, and then every 5–15 min (may cause ↓ BP and respiratory depression); follow standing orders if ↓ BP occurs: terminate infusion; give oxygen by mask; maintain Trendelenburg position; give bolus of crystalloid fluid; notify primary health-care provider.
- Maintain continuous electronic fetal monitoring.
- Assess pain control; notify primary health-care provider if breakthrough pain occurs because dose is ↓ than therapeutic.
- Assess level of sensation and ability to move feet and legs (recovery takes several hours).
- Ensure two people assist with first ambulation after the birth.

Local Infiltration

Insertion of analgesic into perineal tissue; ↓ pain of birth and episiotomy.

Advantages: Technically uncomplicated; does not alter maternal VS or FHR; minimal complications; patient is awake.

Disadvantages: A large volume of agent is needed.

Nursing Care

- Assess effectiveness.
- Ensure thermal injury does not occur if cold application is used to ↓ inflammation.

Spinal Block

Injection of anesthetic into spinal fluid provides anesthesia for cesarean birth and occasionally for vaginal birth with midforceps delivery or vacuum extraction.

Advantages: Ease of administration, immediate onset, patient is awake, smaller medication volume, less shivering, little placental transfer.

Disadvantages: Finite duration, possible severe maternal hypotension and total spinal anesthetic response, may ↓ ability to push.

Nursing Care

- Hypotension: Give 500–1000 mL IV fluids 15–30 min before block.
- Assist to side-lying or sitting position during insertion (patient must remain still); time insertion between contractions.
- Insert urinary retention catheter before cesarean birth.
- Assess VS before insertion and routinely thereafter.
- Move patient with caution because of temporary leg paralysis.
- Vaginal birth: Assist to sitting position for 1–2 min after block so that solution migrates toward sacral area before side-lying; maintain continuous electronic fetal monitoring; encourage bearing down during contractions.
- Cesarean birth: Assist to supine position, with a left lateral tilt, so that cephalad spread of anesthesia occurs.
- Interventions after birth: Maintain bedrest for 6–12 hr; ensure two people assist with first ambulation; assess for urinary retention because sensation and control may not return for 8–12 hr; catheterize as ordered.

General Anesthesia

Induced unconsciousness; requires intubation with cuffed endotracheal tube, ventilation, oxygenation.
Advantages: Total pain relief; optimum operating conditions.
Disadvantages: Patient is not awake; may cause ↓ maternal respirations, vomiting, aspiration, uterine atony; may cause fetal depression.

Nursing Care

- Maintain supine position with left-lateral tilt; insert IV line; give prescribed prophylactic antacid.
- Preoxygenate 3–5 min with 100% oxygen; maintain cricoid ring pressure to occlude esophagus until cuff of endotracheal tube is inflated.
- When extubated, maintain airway; give oxygen; assess VS, ECG, pulse oximetry; keep suction and resuscitative equipment available.

Problems During Labor and Birth

Abruptio Placentae

Partial, marginal, complete separation of placenta from uterine wall >20th week and before birth.
S&S: Painful vaginal bleeding (concealed bleeding if margins are intact), rigid abdomen, shock, nonreassuring fetal signs.

Nursing Care

- Assess for S&S, VS, FHR, bleeding, pain, uterine activity, I&O; serum studies for DIC, PT, PTT.
- Maintain bedrest; give ordered oxygen, IV blood products; prepare for cesarean birth.

Amniotic Fluid Embolism (AFE)

Escape of amniotic fluid into maternal circulation → pulmonary embolus; 80% fatal; ↑ risk of abruptio placentae and hypertonic labor.
S&S: Chest pain, respiratory distress, cyanosis, rapid shock, ↑ anxiety, feelings of doom, cardiovascular collapse, coagulopathy.

Nursing Care
- Assess for S&S of AFE during third and fourth stages of labor; provide aggressive resuscitation if necessary.
- Give ordered IV fluids, PRBC, platelets to control coagulopathy.

Breech Presentation

Fetal presenting part is buttocks, legs, feet, or combination thereof; risk for cord prolapse, fetal hypoxia and injury, maternal injury.
S&S: Identified via Leopold maneuvers; fetal heart tone above umbilicus; meconium without nonreassuring fetal signs; vaginal exam.

Nursing Care
- Assess for S&S; VS; nonreassuring fetal signs; progress of labor.
- Assess birth canal for cord prolapse when membranes rupture.
- Provide pain relief for "back labor" such as massage, IV medications, regional anesthesia.
- Set up for both vaginal and cesarean birth; give emotional support.
- Give prescribed nitroglycerin for rapid uterine relaxation if head becomes trapped.

Premature Rupture of Membranes (PROM)

Ruptured membranes before start of labor.
S&S: Fluid leaking from vagina; amniotic fluid confirmed with fern or nitrazine test.

Nursing Care
- Establish time of rupture; avoid unnecessary vaginal exams.
- Assess for cord compression, FHR, maternal VS, S&S of infection.
- At term and no labor within 12–24 hr: Assist with induction. <37 weeks: Maintain bedrest in hospital; give prescribed prophylactic antibiotics and amnioinfusion of isotonic saline to ↓ risk of cord compression.

Placenta Previa

Low lying: Placenta in close proximity but not covering os; placenta moves away from os as uterus stretches during third trimester (**migrating placenta**).
Marginal: Edge of placenta extends to os and may extend onto os during dilation.
Partial: Os is incompletely covered by placenta.
Total: Placenta completely covers os.
S&S: Third trimester painless bright red bleeding, soft uterus, anemia, ultrasound confirmation.

Nursing Care
- ■ Maintain bedrest; avoid vaginal exams; assess VS, FHR, blood loss.
- ■ Give prescribed IVs and transfusions for excessive blood loss.
- ■ Give betamethasone to ↑ fetal lung maturity; prepare for preterm or cesarean birth.

Precipitous Labor and Birth
Birth with <3-hr labor.
S&S: History of rapid labor; rapid dilation and fetal descent; rapid contractions with ↓ relaxation between each; risk for fetal intracranial hemorrhage and anoxia; risk for maternal laceration and hemorrhage.

Nursing Care
- ■ Remain with patient; encourage panting with contractions.
- ■ Use palm of hand to support fetal head during birth; do not stop birth of fetus.

Prolapsed Cord
Umbilical cord below presenting fetal part.
S&S: Prolonged variable decelerations; baseline bradycardia; observation of cord protruding through cervix.

Nursing Care
- ■ Lift presenting part away from cord gently, which relieves pressure.
- ■ Provide oxygen; elevate patient's hips while on side to ↑ placental perfusion.
- ■ Assess FHR.
- ■ Notify primary health-care provider immediately; prepare for possible cesarean birth.

Ruptured Uterus
Complete or partial separation of uterine tissue from stress of labor or trauma such as scar of previous cesarean birth; fetal mortality >80%; maternal mortality 50%–75%.
S&S: Silent or dramatic; sudden extreme pain; hypotonic or absent contractions; indications of shock such as ↓ BP, ↑ P, pallor, cool clammy skin; may or may not have nonreassuring fetal signs.

Nursing Care
- ■ Prevention: Explore cesarean versus vaginal birth after previous cesarean birth; prevent or limit uterine hyperstimulation.
- ■ After rupture: Give oxygen; prepare for laparotomy for repair or hysterectomy; give ordered blood or blood products; provide emotional support.

Cephalopelvic Disproportion (CPD)

Fetus larger than pelvic diameters; pelvic inlet and/or pelvic outlet diameter narrowed due to small, abnormally shaped or deformed maternal pelvis.
S&S: Prolonged or arrested first or second stage of labor; impaired fetal descent; measurements indicating small pelvic size.

Nursing Care

- Assist with ultrasonography to identify pelvic size.
- Assess for nonreassuring fetal signs; prepare for cesarean birth.

Dystocia

Difficult, painful, or prolonged labor due to conditions such as large fetus, cephalopelvic disproportion, malpresentation, abnormal contractions, multiple fetuses.
Maternal S&S: Exhaustion; extreme pain; ↑ P; contractions with ↑ frequency and ↓ intensity; weak, inefficient, or stopped contractions; cervical trauma.
Fetal S&S: ↑ FHR; nonreassuring signs; fetal demise.

Nursing Care

- Assess for S&S; progress of labor; maternal VS; infection; status of fetus.
- Evaluate response to prescribed oxytocin.
- Provide pain relief measures.
- Assist with ultrasonography to identify pelvic size.
- Have oxygen and resuscitation equipment available.
- Assess neonate for extent of head molding, caput succedaneum, cephalhematoma.

Preterm Labor

Start of labor before EDB due to conditions such as multiple gestation, maternal illness with ↑ T, opioid use, bacteriuria, multiple abortions, pyelonephritis, bacterial vaginitis.
S&S: Contractions between 20–37 weeks with 2 cm dilation and 80% effacement; contractions every 10 min lasting 30 seconds or longer.

Nursing Care

- Maintain lateral recumbent position and quiet environment; provide prescribed tocolytic agents such as ritodrine (Yutopar), terbutaline, $MgSO_4$, indomethacin (Indocin), nifedipine (Procardia) to suppress labor.
- Give prescribed betamethasone (Celestone) to ↓ severity of respiratory distress syndrome 24–48 hr before probable birth.
- Assess FHR, maternal VS, progress of labor.
- Assess for respiratory depression with $MgSO_4$ and tachycardia with terbutaline and ritodrine.

Postpartum: First 6 Weeks After Birth

Maternal Changes During Postpartum

Vital signs: T ≤ 100.4°F during first 24 hr due to exertion and dehydration; BP returns to baseline; P 50–70 bpm for 6–10 days due to ↑ blood volume and ↑ cardiac effort.

Nursing Care
■ Assess VS every 4–8 hr.
■ Complete focused assessment if ↑T (infection), ↑ P, and ↓ BP (hemorrhage).

Fundus
Intermittent contractions return uterus to prepregnant state **(involution):** 12 hr after birth, uterus is up to or 1 fingerbreadth (FB) above umbilicus; descends 1 FB daily; remains firm and in midline; not felt by 7–9 days.

Nursing Care
■ Assess fundal height; massage uterus if boggy but avoid overstimulation.
■ Give prescribed oxytocic.
■ Have patient void if uterus is elevated and deviated to the right of midline.

Teach multipara and breastfeeding mothers that afterpains may accompany involution.

Vaginal Discharge
Red 2–3 days **(lochia rubra);** pinkish brown 3–10 days **(lochia serosa);** whitish yellow 10–21 days **(lochia alba).**

Nursing Care
■ Assess for excessive Peri-Pad saturation (1 pad in 15 min is excessive); check linen under buttocks for blood; assess for S&S of shock.
■ Check lochia for color, amount, clots, odor; should progress from rubra to serosa and finally to alba; teach patient to notify the primary health-care provider if lochia returns to an earlier stage, is excessive, or has an offensive odor.
■ Flush perineum routinely and after toileting; change Peri-Pad after toileting and prn.
■ Teach menstruation returns about 6 weeks when not breastfeeding and 24 weeks when breastfeeding.

Perineum
May be bruised, edematous, episiotomy site if performed.

Nursing Care
■ Assess for hematoma; hemorrhoids; episiotomy site for Redness, Ecchymosis, Edema, Discharge, Approximation (REEDA).

■ Administer cold applications first 24 hr for 15 min on, 45 min off, then warm sitz baths two to four times daily; use anesthetic spray or witch hazel pads.

Breasts
Soft first 2 days; engorgement third to fifth day due to vasodilation.

Nursing Care
■ Encourage wearing supportive bra; use cool applications such as fresh cabbage leaves inside bra.
■ Teach to avoid breast stimulation such as warm shower and stroking.
■ For breastfeeding mother, see Breastfeeding, p. 84 and Nursing Care Related to Breastfeeding, p. 85.
■ For non-breastfeeding mother, see Formula Feeding, p. 87 and Nursing Care Related to Formula Feeding, p. 87.

Circulatory
↑ WBC, ↓ RBC, and ↓ Hb by 4th day; ↑ fibrinogen and ↑ platelets by 1st week; blood volume returns to baseline by 3rd week.

Nursing Care
■ Monitor WBC, RBC, Hb; assess for S&S of thrombophlebitis.
■ Encourage early ambulation and ↑ fluid intake; promote rest.

Urinary
Diuresis in first 24 hr ≥ 1 L urine; ↓ bladder tone, perineal edema, or regional anesthesia may cause retention; urinary retention displaces uterus up and to right of the midline, which may cause impaired involution of the uterus.

Nursing Care
■ Assess I&O, VS.
■ Encourage to void; call primary health-care provider if patient has not voided within 6–8 hr; catheterize if ordered.

Gastrointestinal
↑ Hunger and thirst; ↑ need for protein and calories to support involution and recovery; usually no BMs for several days due to ↓ food during labor, fear of pain (episiotomy, hemorrhoids), ↓ peristalsis during pregnancy.

Nursing Care
■ Provide nutritious diet; assess BMs.
■ Encourage fluids, fiber, and activity to prevent constipation; give prescribed stool softener, suppository, or enema.

Integumentary
↑ diaphoresis in first 24 hr; pigmentation changes such as striae, linea nigra, and darkened areolae begin to fade; separation of rectus abdominis muscles (**diastasis recti**) may be evident.

Nursing Care

- Promote hygiene.

Parenteral Emotional Changes

Phases of Maternal Adjustment

- **Dependent (taking-in):** First 24–48 hr; fatigued but exhilarated; reviews birth process; focuses on self; dependent.
- **Dependent-independent (taking-hold):** Starts on 2nd–3rd day; lasts 10–14 days; begins care of self and infant; eager to learn; still needs nurturing; may have postpartum blues.
- **Interdependent (letting-go):** 3rd–4th weeks; focuses on family as a unit; reasserts relationship with partner; resumes sexual intimacy.

Stages of Transition to Fatherhood

- **Stage 1 (Expectations):** Preconception of future.
- **Stage 2 (Reality):** Realization that expectations not based on fact; feelings of sadness, ambivalence, jealousy, frustration; desire to be more involved.
- **Stage 3 (Transition to mastery):** Conscious decision to take control and become involved with infant.

Nursing Care of Parents

- Encourage attachment and bonding such as eye contact, touching, skin-to-skin contact, rooming-in, infant care.
- Support adjustment to change in role, self-concept.
- Assess interactions with infant; observe for S&S of maternal depression or psychosis (see Tab 5, MENTAL HEALTH, Nursing Care for Patients Who Are Withdrawn, p. 169).
- Notify primary health-care provider if nurse suspects postpartum depression or psychosis.

Problems During Postpartum Period

Cystitis

Bladder infection.

S&S: Pain or burning on urination, fever, frequency, hematuria.

Nursing Care

- Assess for S&S, distention, fundal height; obtain urine C&S.
- ↑ fluids to 3000 mL daily; encourage frequent and complete emptying of bladder.
- Give prescribed antibiotics.

Hematoma

Collection of blood in connective tissue due to episiotomy, prolonged labor, or use of forceps.

S&S: Perineal or rectal pain or pressure; bulging mass in perineum with discoloration; shock.

Nursing Care
- Assess for S&S; apply ice and give analgesics or blood products as ordered.
- Catheterize patient; prepare for surgical ligation or evacuation.

Postpartum Hemorrhage

Bleeding due to uterine atony, laceration, or inversion of uterus during first 24 hr; may be caused by retained placental fragments after first 24 hr.

S&S: ≥ 500 mL vaginal bleeding.

Nursing Care
- Stay with patient; massage fundus; assess for bleeding such as pad counts; monitor changes in VS, Hb, and Hct levels indicating hemorrhage.
- Monitor I&O; provide ordered IV fluids; prepare to give prescribed oxytocin and blood transfusions.

Infection

Reproductive organ infection within 28 days of birth.

S&S: ↑T, chills, pelvic or abdominal pain, vaginal discharge, ↑WBC.

Nursing Care
- Assess for S&S, VS, I&O.
- Enhance comfort, keep warm, encourage 3 L fluid daily; ↑ calorie and protein intake; give prescribed antibiotics.

Pulmonary Embolism

Blood clot in lungs from uterine and/or pelvic veins.

S&S: Dyspnea, ↑ P and R, crackles, cough, chest pain, hemoptysis, anxiety.

Nursing Care
- Assess for S&S of hypoxia; give oxygen; ↑ HOB.
- Give prescribed IV fluids, anticoagulants, streptokinase to dissolve clot(s).
- Notify primary health-care provider immediately.

Subinvolution

Delay of uterus to return to normal size or condition.

S&S: Prolonged or ↑ lochial discharge, excessive bleeding, uterine pain on palpation, large boggy uterus.

Nursing Care

- Assess for S&S, VS, bleeding; perform firm fundal massage.
- Give prescribed oxytocin or methylergonovine (Methergine), antibiotics.
- Prepare for D&C to remove placental fragments.

Thrombophlebitis

Inflammation and clot formation inside a vessel caused by venous stasis and hypercoagulation; confirmed by Doppler ultrasound.

S&S: Pain or tenderness in lower extremity with heat, redness, swelling, positive Homan sign.

Nursing Care

- Assess for S&S; PT; PTT; keep patient on bedrest; elevate leg.
- Give prescribed analgesics and anticoagulants; generally IV heparin 5–7 days followed by warfarin (Coumadin) for 3 months.
- Apply warm, moist heat; do not elicit Homan sign or rub area (may cause embolus); apply antiembolism stockings before getting OOB when ordered.
- Teach safety related to anticoagulants such as use of soft toothbrush and electric razor.

The Newborn

Neonatal Resuscitation Triangle

NEONATAL RESUSCITATION TRIANGLE

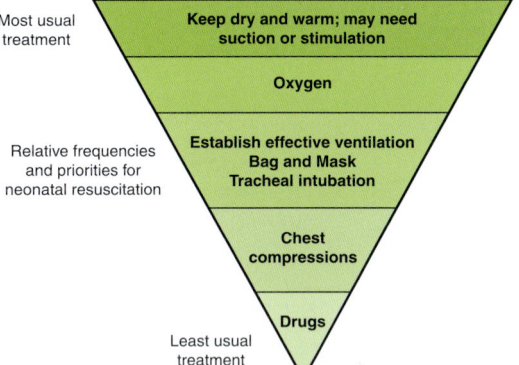

Most usual treatment

Keep dry and warm; may need suction or stimulation

Oxygen

Relative frequencies and priorities for neonatal resuscitation

Establish effective ventilation
Bag and Mask
Tracheal intubation

Chest compressions

Drugs

Least usual treatment

Apgar Score

Sign	Possible Scores			Assessments	
	0	**1**	**2**	**1 min**	**5 min**
Respiratory effort	Absent	Slow, irregular, weak cry	Strong, loud cry		
Heart rate/ pulse	Absent	<100 bpm	>100 bpm		
Muscle tone/ activity	Flaccid	Limited movement, some flexion of extremities	Active movement		
Reflex irritability	None	Grimace, limited cry	Vigorous cry		
Color/ appearance	Pale, blue	Pink torso, blue extremities	Pink torso & extremities		
TOTAL SCORE					

Rating Total Scores
Normal 7–10   4–6 Moderate Depression   0–3 Aggressive Resuscitation

Periods of Reactivity

First Period of Reactivity: First 30–60 min after birth.
Awake, active, strong sucking reflex; HR may be 160–180 bpm and irregular; R may >80 breaths per minute; transient nasal flaring and grunting; no bowel sounds.

Nursing Care
■ Encourage parent-newborn interaction such as eye-to-eye contact, touching, rocking, singing; encourage breastfeeding if desired; provide privacy.

Period of Inactivity/Sleep Phase: Follows first period of reactivity.
Activity ↓; HR and R gradually ↓ to baseline; sleeps 30 min to 4 hr; difficult to awaken; no interest in sucking; bowel sounds audible.

Nursing Care
■ Continue close observation.

Second Period of Reactivity: Awakens from period of inactivity/sleep phase. Alert; lasts 4–6 hr; ↑ response to stimuli; may have ↑ R and HR, apneic episodes, mild cyanosis, mottling; may gag, choke, and regurgitate; may pass meconium stool and first void, sucking, rooting, swallowing indicates readiness for feeding.

Nursing Care
- Maintain airway; stimulate during apneic episodes.
- Encourage breastfeeding if desired; document first void and meconium stool.

Assessment of the Newborn

Normal and Abnormal Characteristics of the Neonate

Weight, Length, Gestational Age	
Expected Characteristics	**Variations/Abnormalities**
Term: Birth 37–42 weeks gestation.	**Intrauterine growth restriction (IUGR):** Fetal weight <10th percentile of expected weight for gestational age.
Appropriate for gestational age (AGA): 10th to 90th percentile for gestational age.	**Preterm:** Birth at <37 weeks gestation.
Birth weight: 2500–4000 g: loss of 10% in first weeks; regained in 10–14 days.	**Post-term:** Birth at >42 weeks gestation.
Crown-to-rump length: 31–35 cm; approximately equal to chest circumference.	**Small for gestational age (SGA):** Birth weight <10th percentile for gestational age.
Head-to-heel length: 48–53 cm.	**Large for gestational age (LGA):** Birth weight >90th percentile for gestational age.
Head circumference: 33–35 cm.	**Low birth weight (LBW):** Birth weight ≤2500 g.
Chest circumference: 30.5–33 cm.	**Very low birth weight (VLBW):** Birth weight ≤1500 g.

Vital Signs	
Expected Characteristics	**Variations/Abnormalities**
Axillary temp: 97.7°F–98.9°F.	**Temp:** Hyperthermia, hypothermia.
Apical pulse: 100–180 bpm after birth, 120–140 bpm when stabilized; murmurs may reflect incomplete closure of fetal shunts.	**Pulse:** *Tachycardia:* >160–180 bpm; *bradycardia:* <80–100 bpm, irregular rhythm, *sinus arrhythmia:* HR ↑ on inspiration and ↑ on expiration.

Vital Signs

Expected Characteristics	Variations/Abnormalities
Respirations: 30–60 bpm; shallow, irregular and abdominal; bilateral bronchial breath sounds. **Blood pressure:** Oscillometric—65/41 mm Hg in arm and calf at 1–3 days of age. **Activity/crying:** May ↑T, P, R, and BP. **Preterm:** ↓ respiratory effort may require oxygen and ventilation; ↓ brown fat and subcutaneous tissue → temperature instability.	**Respirations:** *Tachypnea*: >60 bpm; *apnea*: Absence of breathing >20 sec; nasal flaring, retractions, diminished breath sounds, expiratory grunting, inspiratory stridor, wheezing, crackles. **Blood pressure:** Oscillometric systolic pressure in calf 6–9 mm Hg less than the pressure in an arm may be sign of coarctation of aorta.

Skin

Expected Characteristics	Variations/Abnormalities
Bright red, puffy, smooth skin becomes pink, flaky, and dry by 3rd day. Grayish white, cheesy deposit covering skin **(vernix caseosa).** Fine, downy hair on shoulders, back, and face **(lanugo);** amount ↓ as gestational age ↑. Cyanosis of hands and feet **(acrocyanosis).** Transient mottling **(cutis marmorata)** due to stress, overstimulation, cool environment. Neonatal jaundice after first 24 hr **(physiological jaundice, icterus neonatorum).** **Preterm:** Wrinkled and translucent; abundant lanugo; eyebrows absent; extensive vernix.	Ecchymoses and petechiae. Generalized cyanosis, pallor, mottling, grayness. When lying on side, lower half of body becomes pink and upper half is pale **(harlequin color change).** Progressive jaundice, especially during first 24 hr usually due to Rh or ABO incompatibility. Tenting of skin may indicate dehydration. Light brown spots (café-au-lait spots). Port-wine stain *(nevus flammeus).* Strawberry mark *(nevus vasculosus).* Tiny white papules on cheeks, chin, nose (milia). Flat, deep pink localized areas usually on back of neck *(telangiectatic nevus,* stork bite).

Continued

Skin

Expected Characteristics	Variations/Abnormalities
Post-term: Dry, cracking, parchmentlike skin without vernix or lanugo; greenish tinged skin due to meconium staining.	Irregular areas of deep blue pigmentation usually in sacral or gluteal areas (**Mongolian spots**).

Posture

Expected Characteristics	Variations/Abnormalities
Slight flexion of extremities. Holds head erect momentarily; turns head from side to side when prone; may have brief tremors. **Preterm:** Limp extended limbs; legs abducted.	Limp extended extremities; marked head lag (**hypotonia**). Tremors; twitches; startles easily; arms and hands flexed; legs extended (**hypertonia**). Asymmetric or opisthotonic posturing.

Head Shape and Circumference

Expected Characteristics	Variations/Abnormalities
Circumference: 33–35 cm. **Anterior fontanel:** Diamond-shaped 1–1.75 in. **Posterior fontanel:** Triangle-shaped 0.2–0.4 in. Fontanels are flat, soft, and firm; bulge when crying. Symmetry of face as neonate cries. **Preterm:** Head large compared to chest; small fontanels; hair like matted wool. **Post-term:** Hair may be perfuse.	Molding may occur with vaginal birth; head circumference <10th percentile may indicate microcephaly or >90th percentile may indicate hydrocephalus. Bulging or depressed fontanels when quiet. Widened sutures or fontanels; fused sutures. Asymmetry of face as neonate cries. Diffuse edema of soft scalp tissue that crosses suture line (**caput succedaneum**). Hematoma between periosteum and skull bone (**cephalhematoma**); unilateral and does not cross suture line. **Intracranial hemorrhage:** Muscle twitching; seizures; cyanosis; breathing abnormal; shrill cry.

Eyes

Expected Characteristics	Variations/Abnormalities
Lids edematous. Absence of tears. Blink, corneal, and papillary reflexes present. Funduscopic exam reveals red reflex. Undeveloped fixation on objects. Epicanthal folds in neonates of Asian descent.	Absence of reflexes. Purulent discharge. Epicanthal folds in non-Asians may indicate Down syndrome. Unable to follow bright light. Unable to close one eye with drawing of mouth to one side and inability to wrinkle forehead (**facial palsy**) due to trauma to seventh cranial nerve with vaginal birth or use of forceps.

Ears

Expected Characteristics	Variations/Abnormalities
Startle reflex with loud noises. Ear cartilages formed, pinna flexible; top of pinna on horizontal line with outer canthus of eye. **Preterm:** Ear cartilages undeveloped, ear may fold easily.	Absence of startle reflex in response to noise. Low placement.

Nose

Expected Characteristics	Variations/Abnormalities
Compressed and bruised. Nostrils patent with thin white discharge; sneezing.	Nonpatent nostrils. Purulent or copious nasal discharge. Flaring of nares.

Mouth

Expected Characteristics	Variations/Abnormalities
Intact, arched palate with uvula in midline. Frenulum of tongue and upper lip. Extrusion, gag, rooting, and sucking reflexes present.	Incomplete closure of lip (**cleft lip**); incomplete closure of plate or roof of mouth (**cleft palate**). Enlarged, protruding tongue; profuse salivation may indicate Down syndrome.

Continued

Mouth

Expected Characteristics	Variations/Abnormalities
Minimal salivation. Vigorous cry.	Cry: Absent, weak, high-pitched. White patches on oral membranes and tongue **(candidiasis, thrush)**.

Neck

Expected Characteristics	Variations/Abnormalities
Short, thick with multiple skin folds. Tonic neck reflex present.	Excessive skin folds. Absence of tonic neck reflex.

Chest

Expected Characteristics	Variations/Abnormalities
Anteroposterior and lateral diameters equal. Xiphoid process evident. Bilateral areola and breast bud tissue 0.5–1 cm; breast tissue ↑ as gestational age ↑. Mild sternal retractions on inspiration. **Preterm:** Absent or ↓ breast tissue.	Depressed sternum, funnel chest **(pectus excavatum)**; pigeon chest **(pectus carinatum)**. Wide-spaced nipples, extra nipples **(supernumerary nipples)**. Milky discharge from breast **(witch's milk)**. Marked sternal retractions during inspiration. Asymmetric chest expansion.

Abdomen

Expected Characteristics	Variations/Abnormalities
Umbilical cord: Bluish white; two arteries and one vein. Presence of bowel sounds. **Liver:** Palpable 2–3 cm below right costal margin. **Spleen:** Tip palpable left costal margin by 1 week. **Kidneys:** Palpable 1–2 cm above umbilicus. **Preterm:** ↓ Bowel sounds.	Presence of one artery in cord. Umbilical hernia obvious when crying. Cord bleeding or hematoma. Gap between recti muscles **(diastasis recti)**. Abdominal distention; absent bowel sounds. Visible peristaltic waves. Enlarged liver or spleen.

Back and Rectum

Expected Characteristics	Variations/Abnormalities
Spine intact. Trunk incurvation **(Galant)** reflex present. Patent anal opening. Passage of meconium within 24 hr. Anal constriction when touched **(anal wink)**.	External saclike protrusion along spinal column **(spina bifida)**. Dimple with tuft of hair along spine **(pilonidal cyst)**; may indicate underlying spina bifida occulta. No trunk incurvation reflex. No anal opening **(imperforate anus)**. No meconium passed within 36 hr.

Extremities

Expected Characteristics	Variations/Abnormalities
Symmetrical with full ROM; 10 fingers and toes; feet flat; creases on anterior 2/3 of sole. **Preterm:** Fine wrinkles; flexing of hand toward forearm creates angle that ↓ with ↑ in gestational age **(square window sign)**. Elbow in relation to midline when arm is drawn across chest: The farther the elbow passes the midline, the ↓ gestational age **(scarf sign)**. **Post-term:** Long fingernails.	Extra digits; fused/webbed digits; palmar simian crease may indicate Down syndrome. ↓ ROM; fractures of clavicle, humerus, or femur; signs of paralysis. Audible click on flexion and abduction of hips **(Ortolani sign)** and unequal gluteal or leg folds may indicate developmental dysplasia of the hip. Fixed plantar flexion with medial deviation **(clubfoot, talipes equinovarus)**. Flaccid arm with elbow extended and hand internally rotated **(Duchenne-Erb paralysis)** due to birth trauma.

Male Genitalia

Expected Characteristics	Variations/Abnormalities
Urethral opening at tip of penis. Scrotum developed; pendulous, multiple rugae, and contains testes. May be unable to retract foreskin.	Urethra opens on ventral surface **(hypospadias)** or dorsal surface **(epispadias)**. Ventral curvature of penis **(chordee)**. Fluid in scrotum **(hydrocele)**.

Continued

Male Genitalia	
Expected Characteristics	**Variations/Abnormalities**
Urination within 24 hr. **Preterm:** Scrotum undeveloped.	Testes not palpable. Ambiguous genitalia. No urination within 24 hr.

Female Genitalia	
Expected Characteristics	**Variations/Abnormalities**
Urethral opening between clitoris and vagina. Labia majora developed; nonprominent clitoris. Urination within 24 hr. **Preterm:** Labia majora incompletely developed; clitoris prominent.	Enlarged clitoris with urethral opening at tip. Fused labia; no vaginal opening. Blood-tinged or mucoid vaginal discharge **(pseudomenstruation)**. Ambiguous genitalia. No urination within 24 hr.

Reflexes in the Neonate

Reflex Name	Physical Response
Babinski	When stimulating outer sole of foot from heel upward and across ball of foot toward large toe, the large toe dorsiflexes and toes flare; persists 1 yr.
Blink	When startled or quick movement is made toward eye, eyelids close; persists for life.
Corneal	When cornea is directly stimulated, eyelids close; persists for life.
Crawl	When placed on abdomen, arms and legs make crawling motions; persists 6 weeks.
Extrusion	When tongue is touched, tongue moves forward out through the lips; persists 4 months.
Gag	When stimulating posterior pharynx, choking occurs; persists for life.
Grasp	When palm **(palmar reflex)** or sole of foot **(plantar reflex)** is stimulated at base of digits, fingers and toes flex in griplike motion; persists 3 months and 8 months, respectively.

Reflex Name	Physical Response
Moro (startle)	When startled by noise or jarring, arms extend and abduct with fingers forming a C while knees and hips flex slightly, arms return to chest in an embracing motion; persists 3–4 months.
Step (dance)	When supported under both arms with feet against firm surface, feet will make stepping movements; persists 3–4 weeks.
Pupillary	When retina stimulated by light, pupil constricts; persists for life.
Rooting	When touching cheek or lips, head turns toward touch and mouth opens in attempt to suck; lasts 3–4 months, may persist 1 yr.
Sucking	When object touches lips or is placed in mouth, sucking is attempted; persists through infancy.
Tonic neck (fencing)	When supine with head turned to one side, extremities on same side straighten and extremities on opposite side flex; persists 3–4 months.
Trunk incurvation (Galant)	When stroking infant's back alongside spine, hips move toward stimulated side; persists 4 weeks.

Nursing Care of the Newborn

■ **Patent airway:** Suction mouth and then nasal passages; insert bulb syringe or DeLee catheter alongside of mouth to avoid gag reflex; use side-lying position with roll behind back.

■ **Identification:** Apply matching ID bracelets to newborn and mother with name, sex, date, and time of birth, ID number (significant others may also wear bracelets); obtain newborn footprint on form with mother's fingerprints, name, date, time of birth; identify before mother and newborn are separated.

■ **Body temperature:** Dry baby thoroughly; put on a cap; place on mother's abdomen; cover with warm blanket in an Isolette or unclothed under radiant warmer; assess temperature (use axillary or ThermoProbe) every hr until stable; rectal route contraindicated. Newborn is unable to shiver and breaks down brown fat to produce energy for warmth; stress increases need for oxygen and upsets acid-base balance.

- **Eye prophylaxis:** Insert ophthalmic antibiotic such as 0.5% erythromycin or 1% tetracycline into lower conjunctiva of each eye; prevents gonorrheal or chlamydial infection of eyes **(ophthalmia neonatorum)** contracted during vaginal birth; insert after parent-newborn attachment is facilitated.
- **Vitamin K:** Give IM dose of vitamin K (0.5–1 mg phytonadione) to promote normal clotting; vitamin K is produced in the GI tract when bacterial formation occurs after ingesting breast milk or formula, usually by 8th day.
- **Umbilical cord:** Clamp for 24 hr until cord is dry; assess for bleeding or infection; clean cord with soap and water after each diaper change; place diaper below umbilical cord stump; continue care until cord falls off naturally in about 10–14 days. Teach parents related principles.
- **Bathing:** Bathe with warm water and mild soap to remove amniotic fluid, blood, vaginal secretions, skin residue; keep environment warm and draft-free to ↓ chilling; dry and swaddle infant; sponge bathe daily—tub bath after cord falls off and circumcision is healed usually within 2 weeks. Teach parents related principles.
- **Circumcision:** Assess for swelling; redness and bleeding every 30 min for 2 hr, then every 2 hr for 24 hr, then with each diaper change; assess urination (<6 diapers a day may indicate edema is occluding urethra); change dressing as ordered such as 3 times on first day and then daily for 3 days; apply petroleum jelly with or without gauze; avoid disrupting yellowish exudate that appears on second day, as this is part of the healing process; apply diaper loosely to ↓ pressure and friction; give prescribed analgesic. Teach parents related principles. Support the desire of parents who are Jewish to have the circumcision conducted by a mohel during a religious ceremony on the 8th day of life (Bris, Brit Milah Ceremony).

Infant Feeding

Breastfeeding

Maternal Benefits

Increases attachment; releases oxytocin, promoting uterine contraction and involution (lochia flow may ↑); extends anovulation beyond 4–6 weeks; contraception should be discussed with primary health-care provider if desired; convenient and economical; ↓ risk of breast and ovarian cancer.

Newborn Benefits

Increases attachment; optimum nutritional value for first 6 months of age (advocated by the American Academy of Pediatrics); provides immunological components such as passive immunity via IgE, IgM, and IgA immunoglobulins, macrophages, leukocytes, lymphocytes, and neutrophils; ↓ incidence of morbidity and mortality.

Contraindications

Mother: HIV positive (except in developing countries where HIV is prevalent because the benefits outweigh the risk); active TB; opioid addiction; breast abnormalities from trauma, burns, radiation; chronic disease that interferes with lactation or maternal status; taking medications excreted in breast milk that are harmful to infant; inadequate maternal fluid and/or nutrition intake.

Newborn: Anomalies that prevent ingestion such as cleft palate or inborn errors of metabolism that cause negative response to breast milk; preterm infant may not have energy to suck; breast milk may be given by bottle or gastric tube.

Nursing Care Related to Breastfeeding

Initial Assessment

■ Determine mother's desire to breastfeed, level of anxiety, condition of nipples, maternal and infant physical status, family support.

Teach Self–Breast Care

■ Cleanse breasts with water daily; avoid soap and alcohol because of drying effect.

■ Wear a supportive brassiere day and night.

■ Wear nursing pads to absorb leaking milk; allow nipples to air-dry several times a day.

Teach Breastfeeding Techniques

■ Begin breastfeeding as soon as possible, preferably in birthing room.

■ Offer breast every 2–3 hr or on demand; infant feeding cues include sucking movements and hand-to-mouth motions.

■ Assume comfortable position such as semi-reclining or sitting; place infant with entire body facing breast using cradle, side-lying, or football hold.

■ Alternate starting breast and use both breasts at each feeding to ↑ milk production.

■ Stimulate rooting reflex and direct nipple and entire areola into open mouth above tongue **(latching-on).** Nipple stimulation or emotional response to infant precipitates tingling sensation in breast as milk enters ducts and is secreted from breasts **(let-down reflex).**

■ Burp infant during and after feeding; rub or pat back while infant sits on mother's lap, flexed forward to allow for assessment of airway.

■ Place in infant seat or supine with head of mattress slightly elevated after feeding to ↓ regurgitation, reflux, and SIDS.

■ Pump breast milk and store for future use if desired; refrigerate for 72 hr or freeze for ≤ 6 months; date each bottle and use oldest first; do not warm in microwave oven.

- Evaluate maternal and neonate response to breastfeeding.
- Document knowledge and demonstration of effective breast care, breast pumping, and breastfeeding.

Problems Encountered With Breastfeeding

Breast Engorgement
Breasts are swollen, hard, hot, tender and may be dry and red due to vascular congestion before secreting milk; usually occurs 3–5 days postpartum.

Nursing Care
- Encourage breastfeeding every 2 hr and to empty breasts entirely by pumping if necessary; otherwise back pressure on full milk glands ↓ milk production.
- Apply ice between feedings 15 min on and 45 min off; avoid heat because it will ↑ vascular congestion.

Inverted Nipples
Nipples are below surface of surrounding skin.

Nursing Care
- Wear breast shield to draw nipple out.
- Use electric breast pump before attempting latching-on.
- Apply ice, tug and roll nipple with hands before feeding.

Sore or Cracked Nipples
Nipple irritation resulting in discomfort or pain.

Nursing Care
- Alternate infant position; use less-sore nipple first; use breast shield.
- Ensure infant has the areola and not just the nipple in the mouth.
- Apply ice before feeding to ↑ nipple erectness and ↓ soreness OR breast massage and warm compress before feeding to ↑ let-down reflex.
- Analgesic 1 hr before feeding to ↓ soreness.
- Apply breast milk to nipples and air-dry at end of feeding.

Mastitis
Infection of breast; often occurs 2–3 weeks after birth when breastfeeding; flu-like clinical manifestations; ↑T; local heat and swelling; discomfort or pain.

Nursing Care
- Assess for S&S.
- Apply heat or cold as ordered; give prescribed analgesics and antibiotics.
- Encourage continued lactation or use of breast pump every 4 hr; suggest use of supportive bra; teach hand and breast hygiene.

Formula Feeding (Bottle-Feeding)

Benefits
More freedom for mother; permits feeding by significant others; allows for accurate assessment of intake; special formulas can be given for infants with allergies or inborn errors of metabolism; appropriate for infants with congenital anomalies such as cleft palate.

Contraindications
Cost of formula and equipment; lack of time or ability to prepare, store, and refrigerate bottles of formula; potential for contaminated water supply.

Nursing Care Related to Formula Feeding

Teach Regarding Formulas
- Formula should yield 110–130 calories and 130–200 mL of fluid/kg of body weight.
- From birth to 2 months 6–8 feedings of 2–4 oz of formula may be ingested in 24 hr.
- Formula may be ready-to-feed, concentrated, or powder; sterilization may be necessary if water source is questionable; prepare 1 day supply at a time and discard if not used within 48 hr.
- Regular cow's milk not appropriate <12 months of age because of ↑ protein and ↑ calcium and less vitamin C, iron, and carbohydrates than breast milk.

Teach Formula-Feeding Techniques
- Warm bottle by placing it in warm water; never use microwave oven.
- Sprinkle a few drops on wrist to test temperature.
- Offer bottle every 2½–4 hr or on demand.
- Start with 3 oz in each bottle.
- Always hold infant because propping bottle may cause aspiration.
- Support entire length of body with head elevated and attempt eye-to-eye contact.
- Enlarge nipple hole size for infant with ↓ sucking reflex or ↓ energy if advised by primary health-care provider.
- Keep nipple filled with formula to ↓ air ingestion; burp during and after feeding.
- Place in infant seat or supine with head of mattress slightly elevated after feeding to↓ regurgitation, reflux, and SIDS.
- Discard unused formula with each feeding.
- Evaluate maternal and neonate response to formula feeding.
- Document knowledge and demonstration of effective formula preparation and feeding techniques.

Problems Encountered With Formula Feeding

Overdilution of formula → inadequate gain in weight.
Underdilution of formula → excess gain in weight.
Infant may not tolerate fats or carbohydrates found in formula.
Bacterial contamination during preparation and storage may occur.

* From Rubin, R. (1961). Basic maternal behavior. *Nursing Outlook* 9, 683–686.
** From Henderson, A., and Brouse, A. (1991). The Experiences of New Fathers.
During the First Three Weeks of Life. *J of Adv Nursing*, 16 (3), 293–298.

Neurological Problems
  Neural Tube Defects
  Hydrocephalus
  Anencephaly
  Cerebral Palsy (CP)
  Cognitive Impairment (Mental Retardation)
Chromosome Disorders
  Turner Syndrome
  Klinefelter Syndrome
  Trisomy 21 (Down Syndrome)
Skeletal Malformations
  Clubfoot (Talipes Equinovarus) and Developmental Dysplasia of the Hip (DDH)
  Scoliosis
Juvenile Idiopathic Arthritis
Infections and Infestations
Viral Infections
Integumentary System Problems
  Atopic Dermatitis (Eczema)
  Burns
Poisoning

Age-Appropriate Vital Sign Ranges

	Heart Rate	Respirations	Blood Pressure
Newborn	80–180	30–60	60–80/30–60
Toddler	80–110	24–32	90–100/50–65
School-Age	60–110	18–26	95–110/55–70
Adolescent	50–90	16–20	110–120/60–80
Adult	60–100	12–20	110–140/60–90

Immunization Schedule—United States, 2012

Recommended Immunization Schedule for Persons Age 0–6 Years

Vaccine	Birth	1 month	2 months	4 months	6 months	12 months	15 months	18 months	19-23 months	2-3 years	4-6 years
Hepatitis B	Hep B	Hep B			Hep B						
Rotavirus			RV	RV	RV						
Diphtheria, Tetanus, Pertussis			DTaP	DTaP	DTaP		DTaP				DTaP
Haemophilus influenzae type b			Hib	Hib	Hib	Hib					
Pneumococcal			PCV	PCV	PCV	PCV				PPSV	
Inactivated Poliovirus			IPV	IPV	IPV						IPV
Influenza					Influenza (Yearly)						
Measles, Mumps, Rubella						MMR					MMR
Varicella						Varicella					Varicella
Hepatitis A						HepA (2 doses)				HepA Series	
Meningococcal						MCV4					

■ Recommended range for all

■ Certain high-risk groups

■ Range for all children & certain high-risk groups

Recommended Immunization Schedule for Persons Age 7–18 Years

For those who fall behind or start late, see the schedule below and the catch-up schedule

Age Vaccine	7–10 years	11–12 years	13–18 years
Diphtheria, Tetanus, Pertussis	1 dose (if indicated)	1 dose	1 dose (if indicated)
Human Papillomavirus		3 doses	Complete 3-dose series
Meningococcal		Dose 1	Booster at 16
Influenza	Influenza (Yearly)		
Pneumococcal	PPSV		
Hepatitis A	Complete 2-dose series		
Hepatitis B	Complete 3-dose series		
Inactivated Poliovirus	Complete 3-dose series		
Measles, Mumps, Rubella	Complete 2-dose series		
Varicella	Complete 2-dose series		

Legend:
- ■ Range of recommended ages
- ■ Catch-up immunization
- ■ Certain high-risk groups

Nursing Care Related to Administration of Immunizations

- Assess for contraindications: High fever; acquired passive immunity (maternal antibodies, blood transfusions, immunoglobulin); immunosuppression; previous allergic response; pregnancy—measles, mumps, and rubella vaccinations.
- Follow schedule.
- Use appropriate-length needle to reach muscle to ↓ local reactions.
- Use age-appropriate muscle—vastus lateralis or ventrogluteal for infants; deltoid may be used ≥18 months.
- Apply topical anesthetic spray at injection site; inject slowly.
- Teach side effects: Systemic—low-grade temperature; local—tenderness, erythema, and swelling; behavioral—drowsiness, irritability, and anorexia.

Growth and Development

Infant: 1–12 Months

Physical
- Weight triples; chest approaches head circumference; 6–8 teeth.
- Turns from abdomen to back by 5 months and back to abdomen by 6 months.
- Sits by 7 months.
- Crawls, pulls self up, and uses pincer grasp by 9 months.
- Walks holding on by 11 months.

Psychosocial
- Task: Development of trust that → faith and optimism; support task by meeting needs immediately.
- Oral stage: Provide pacifier for comfort and to meet oral needs.
- Egocentric; smiles and focuses on bright objects by 2 months; laughs by 4 months; separation anxiety begins by 4–8 months; fears strangers by 6–8 months—provide consistent caregiver.
- May have security object—keep object available.

Cognitive
- Sensorimotor phase; reflexes replaced by voluntary activity.
- Beginning understanding of cause and effect by 1–4 months.
- Knows objects moved out of sight still exist (**object permanence**) by 9–10 months.

Language
- Crying signals displeasure first 6 months.
- Babbles by 3 months; imitates sounds by 6 months; reacts to simple commands by 9 months; says one word by 10 months; says 3 to 5 words and understands 100 by 12 months.

Play
- Plays alone (solitary play); involves own body; becomes more interactive and shows toy preferences by 3–6 months; involves sensorimotor skills by 6–12 months—ensure play is interactive, recreational, and educational.
- Toys: Must be large enough to prevent aspiration; should be simple because of short attention span; use black and white or bright mobiles, stuffed animals, rattles, teething rings, push-pull toys, blocks, and books with textures.

Injury Prevention
- *Suffocation/aspiration:* Avoid pillows, excessive bedding, tucked-in blankets, baby powder, propping bottles, latex balloons, buttons, plastic bags; use cribs with stationary side rails, corner posts no higher than 1/16 inch above end panel, and vertical slats $\leq 2\frac{3}{8}$ inch apart.
- *Motor vehicle:* Use rear-facing car seat with five-point harness until child exceeds height and weight indicated by manufacturer (usually 22–35 pounds); do not leave in car unattended.
- *Falls:* Supervise when on raised surface; place gates at top and bottom of stairs; use restraints with infant seat, high chair, walker, or swing.
- *Poisoning:* Store agents in high, locked cabinet; avoid secondhand smoke; keep poison control center number by telephone.
- *Burns:* Set water heater at $\leq 120°F$; test water before bath; use bathtub not sink for baths; avoid exposure to sun; do not use microwave to warm bottle; put inserts in electric outlets, and install smoke and heat detectors throughout house.
- *Drowning:* Supervise when in or near water such as bathtub, toilet, bucket, pool, lake; keep toilet lid down with safety lock; know CPR.

Reaction to Illness, Hospitalization, Pain
- Before 6 months, recognizes pain; not emotionally troubled by intrusive procedures.
- Signs and Symptoms (S&S) of pain: high-pitched cry, irritability, tearing, stiff posture, fisting, brows lowered and drawn together, eyes tightly closed, mouth open, difficulty sleeping and eating.
- Nursing care:
  - Meet needs immediately to ↑ trust.
  - Provide nipple dipped in sucrose solution during painful procedure; administer prescribed pain medication.

Nursing Care of Infants
■ After 6 months see information under Toddler: 12–36 Months following.

Toddler: 12–36 Months

Physical
■ ↓ growth rate; birth weight quadruples by 2.5 yr.
■ Anterior fontanel closed by 18 months; chest > head circumference.
■ ↓ appetite **(physiological anorexia)**; 20 teeth.
■ ↓ naps; daytime bowel and bladder control at 2 yr and night control by 3–4 yr.
■ ↑ taste preferences; walks by 14 months; runs by 18 months.
■ Mastery of gross and fine motor movements.

Psychosocial
■ Task: Autonomy → self-control—encourage independence.
■ Anal stage of development.
■ Differentiates self from others; notes sex role differences; explores own body.
■ Withstands short periods of delayed gratification and parental separation.
■ Negativistic—give choices, avoid frustration, provide for safety while ignoring tantrum.
■ Needs routines and may suck thumb for comfort—support routines.
■ May fear sleep, engines, and animals; may have a security object.
■ Sibling rivalry with newborn—supervise interaction, give individual attention, include in newborn care, provide doll for imitative play.

Cognitive
■ Continuation of sensorimotor phase.
■ Preconceptional thought by 2–4 yr; beginning of memory.
■ ↑ sense of time; asking why and how by 2 yr; magical thinking.
■ ↑ concept of ownership (mine); beginning conscience.

Language
■ Comprehension; four to six words by 15 months; ≥10 at 18 months; >300 at 2 yr.
■ Talks incessantly; sentences by 2 yr.

Play
■ Plays alongside, not with, other children **(parallel play)**; imitative.
■ Types of play: Interactive, recreational, and educational.
■ Interactions: Alone, peers, adults.
■ Environments: Home, park, preschool.
■ Activities: Quiet, active, structured, unstructured—provide varieties of play.

Toys:

- **Physical:** Push-pull objects; use pounding board, pedal-propelled toys; balls.
- **Social/creative:** Telephone, dolls, safe kitchen utensils, dress-up, trucks.
- **Fine-motor skills:** Crayons, nesting blocks, tactile such as finger paints and clay.
- **Cognitive:** Simple puzzles, picture books, appropriate TV programs and videos.

Injury Prevention

- ↑ risk due to desire for independence, lack of judgment, immature physical abilities.
- *Motor vehicle:* Use forward-facing seat with a five-point harness for all children who have exceeded height and weight recommended for rear-facing seat even if under 1 yr of age; use forward-facing seat until height child exceeds belt-positioning booster seat; do not leave in car unattended.
- *Drowning:* Supervise when in or near water; fence or cover pool and hot tub; toilet seat down with safety lock; know CPR.
- *Burns:* Turn handles of pots to back of stove; front guards on radiators, space heaters, fireplaces; keep appliance cords, candles, and iron out of reach.
- *Poisoning:* Store agents in high, locked cabinet; avoid secondhand smoke; keep poison control center number by telephone.
- *Suffocation/aspiration:* Avoid foods that may occlude airway such as nuts, grapes, hot dogs, hard candy; keep garage door openers inaccessible; avoid toy boxes with heavy hinged lids, clothing with drawstrings, appliances that cannot be opened from inside.
- *Bodily damage:* Avoid running with objects in mouth and jumping near doors or furniture with glass; hold pointed objects downward; keep tools and firearms in locked cabinet; keep away from lawnmowers; teach to never go with a stranger or allow inappropriate touching.

Reaction to Illness, Hospitalization, Pain

- Fears punishment, the unknown, separation, immobilization, isolation.
- Altered rituals ↑ stress; regresses when anxious.
- Stages of separation anxiety:
- **Protest:** Inconsolable crying and rejects others.
- **Despair:** Flat affect, unresponsive to stimuli, altered sleep, ↑ appetite.
- **Detachment/denial:** Lack of preference for parents; friendly to all.
- **S&S of pain:** Expresses pain in a word (ow), regresses, clings to parent, cries.
- **Nursing care:**
- Provide consistent routines and caregiver.
- Encourage parent to stay with child when possible.
- Ignore regression while praising appropriate behavior.

- Provide massage.
- Use distraction.
- Administer thermotherapy and medications as prescribed.

Preschooler: 3–5 Years

Physical
- Average ↑ weight 5 pounds per year; ↑ height 2.5–3 inches per year.
- ↑ immune responses.
- ↑ strength; refinement of gross and fine motor skills.
- Dresses and washes self; skips, hops, jumps rope, skates, holds pencil and utensils with fingers; uses scissors by 5 yr.
- Potential for amblyopia by 4–6 yr—assess for nonbinocular vision **(strabismus)**.

Psychosocial
- Task: Development of initiative promotes direction and purpose which encourage endeavors.
- Oedipal stage of psychosexual development; attaches to parent of opposite sex while identifying with same-sex parent—encourage imitative and imaginative play; begin informal sex education.
- May have imaginary friend; selfish; impatient; exaggerates.
- Beginning morality (difference between right and wrong); personality developed by 5 yr.

Cognitive
- ↑ preconceptual thought; intuitive thought by 4–5 yr.
- ↑ readiness for learning; curious about immediate world.
- Considers another's views; understands past, present, and future by 5 yr.

Language
- ↑ complexity; uses all parts of speech; asks meaning of new words.
- Knows 900 words by 3 yr; 1500 by 4 yr; 2100 by 5 yr.
- Stuttering and stammering common during 2–4 yr.

Play
- Group play without rigid rules **(associative play)**.
- Physical, manipulative, imitative, imaginary play; ↑ sharing by 5 yr.
- Toys:
  - *Physical:* Playground, uses sports equipment, bicycles.
  - *Social/creative:* Dress-up, puppets, villages.
  - *Fine motor skills:* Construction sets, simple musical instruments, craft projects.
  - *Cognitive:* Computer games with numbers and letters, simple board games, activity books.

Injury Prevention

- Similar to toddler but not as significant due to ↑ fine and gross motor skills, coordination, balance; ↑ awareness of danger and parental rules.
- Teach safety habits: Look both ways, wear helmets, play in yard or play-ground; parents should set example of acceptable behavior.
- Motor vehicle injuries: Use forward-facing seat until child exceeds recommended height and weight (usually 20–40 pounds) and then use belt-positioning booster seat; do not leave in car unattended.
- Teach difference between acceptable and unacceptable touching and to tell parent or a person they trust if they are being touched inappropriately.

Reaction to Illness, Hospitalization, Pain

- Fears intrusive procedures, pain, punishment, rejection, bodily harm, castration, darkness more than separation.
- S&S of pain: Crying, biting, hitting, kicking.
- Death viewed as temporary.

Nursing Care

- Explain and demonstrate what may be experienced to ↓ anxiety.
- Visit hospital before elective procedure or surgery.
- Support therapeutic play with dolls, medical equipment; use distraction, massage; administer thermotherapy and medications as prescribed.

School-Age Child: 6–12 Years

Physical

- Bone precedes muscular development.
- Average ↑ height 2 inches per year; ↑ weight 4.5–6.5 lb per year; girls pass boys in height and weight by 12 yr.
- Permanent teeth begin with front teeth; puberty begins earlier in females (about 10 yr) than males (about 12 yr).

Psychosocial

- Task: Achievement of industry ← → personal and interpersonal competence—recognize accomplishments, avoid comparisons.
- Latent stage of psychosexual development; ↑ egocentricity.
- Identifies with peers of same sex by 6–10 yr; beginning interest in opposite sex by 10–12 yr.
- Develops intrinsic motivation (mastery, self-satisfaction).
- Behaves according to set norms; develops self-image, body image.

Cognitive

- Concrete operations, inductive reasoning, beginning logic by 7–11 yr.
- Grasps concepts of conservation.
- Classifies, serializes, tells time, and reads.

Language
- Vocabulary and comprehension expand.
- Adult speech well established by 9–12 yr.

Play
- ↑ ego mastery, conformity in play, fanatic about rules.
- ↑ peer relationships such as team sports and clubs.
- Collections are more selective; ↑ complexity of board games.
- Engages in hero worship—promote positive role model.

Injury Prevention
- ↑ risk-taking behaviors due to ↑ physical abilities, ↓ parental supervision, poor judgment; more injuries in boys than girls.
- Motor vehicle: Teach pedestrian skills; play in park, not street; use belt-positioning booster seat when child exceeds recommended weight and height for forward-facing seat; use booster seat until vehicle seat belt fits properly (usually 4 feet 9 inches in height and between 8 and 12 yr of age); then use vehicle-provided lap and shoulder seat belts; all children under the age of 13 should sit in the rear seat.
- Bodily damage: Wear eye, mouth, and ear protection with sports; supervise climbing and gymnastics.
- Teach to go to school nurse if experiencing bullying, sexual harassment, or abuse; never go with a stranger.
- Toxic substances: Role-play saying *no* to tobacco, drugs, alcohol.

Reaction to Illness, Hospitalization, Pain
- Fears the unknown, loss of control, dependency, disfigurement, death.
- Typifies death as bogeyman; has realistic concept of death by 9–10 yr.
- S&S of pain: Attempts to cooperate or stays rigid for painful procedures; may cry, yell, resist; clenched fists, gritted teeth, closed eyes, wrinkled forehead.
- Nursing care:
  - Place with age-appropriate roommate; support visits from peers, doing schoolwork.
  - Provide privacy for activities of daily living and procedures.
  - Permit wearing underpants; allow touching of equipment; provide choices; praise attempts at cooperation; encourage expression of feelings; never belittle regression, resistance, crying.
  - Use pain scale, distraction, guided imagery, thought stopping, soothing music, massage; administer prescribed thermotherapy and medications for pain.

Adolescent: 12–21 Yr

- Early adolescence (11–14 yr): Changes of puberty and reaction to changes.
- Middle adolescence (15–17 yr): Transition to peer group identification.
- Late adolescence (18–21 yr): Transition into adulthood.

Physical
- Uncoordinated as linear exceeds muscular growth; ↑ strength, especially males.
- Male puberty 12–16 yr: Enlargement of scrotum, testes, and penis; pubic, axillary, facial, body hair; nocturnal emissions, mature spermatozoa; voice deepens; 95% of height by 15 yr.
- Female puberty 10–14 yr: Development of breasts, pubic, axillary hair; first menstruation **(menarche)**; ovulation about 12 months after menarche; 95% of height by menarche.

Psychosocial
- Task: Developing sense of identity → positive self-concept and body.
- Feels omnipotent; behavior motivated by peer group.
- Resists enforcement of discipline.
- Desires independence but may avoid responsibilities.
- ↑ interest in appearance; ↑ interest in sex (experimentation); forms intimate relationships (opposite sex if heterosexual; same sex if homosexual).

Cognitive
- Formal operational thought; capable of abstract, conceptual, hypothetical thinking; comprehends satire and double meanings.
- ↑ learning through inference vs. repetition and imitation.
- Difficulty accepting another viewpoint; idealistic.
- Develops personal value systems **(value autonomy)**.

Language
- ↑ vocabulary and reading comprehension.
- Experiments with language, uses jargon.

Play
- Individual and team sports provide exercise; ↑ social and personal development; and permit experience of competition, teamwork, and conflict resolution.
- Follows rules of complex games such as Monopoly and chess.

Injury Prevention
- Risk-taking due to feelings of omnipotence, independence, or to impress peers.
- *Motor vehicle:* Assess level of responsibility and ability to resist peer pressure; set limits on driving; encourage wearing lap and shoulder seat belt.

- *Sports*: Encourage warming up and cooling down, playing within abilities, wearing protective gear.
- *Suicide and homicide:* Males more than females; related to economic deprivation, family dysfunction, availability of firearms; assess risk due to frustration, deprivation, aggression, depression, social isolation; lock up firearms.
- Teach to go to school nurse if experiencing bullying, sexual harassment or abuse.
- *Sexually transmitted infections (STI):* May not seek medical care due to lack of S&S, misinformation, guilt, shame, fear; teach sex education and STI prevention such as abstinence or ↓ number of partners, use of condoms; role-play resisting peer pressure.

Reaction to Illness, Hospitalization, Pain
- Similar to school-age child; ↑ need for independence, privacy, body integrity.
- Fear of disfigurement or ↓ function.
- ↓ need for parental visits, but separation from peers may be traumatic.
- S&S of pain: Physical pain tolerated; stoicism important among males; clenched fist, gritting teeth, self-splinting; ↓ interest, concentration; has realistic concept of death but emotionally may be unable to accept it.
- Nursing care:
  - Use distraction, music, massage.
  - Encourage peer relationships.

Genitourinary Malformations

Exstrophy of the Bladder

- Absence of portion of abdominal and bladder walls causing eversion of bladder through opening.

Signs and Symptoms
- Presence of defect; leaking of urine; urine smell due to leaking.
- Associated defects: Pubic bone malformation, inguinal hernia, epispadias, undescended testes or short penis in males, cleft clitoris or absent vagina in females.

Treatment
- Surgical repair.

Nursing Care
Infant
- Cover bladder with clear plastic wrap or thin film dressing without adhesive.
- Apply prescribed protective barrier to protect skin from urine.
- Assess intake and output (I&O) and drainage from bladder or ureteral drainage tubes.
- Assess bowel function if surgery included resection of intestine.
- Care after surgery for penile lengthening; chordee release; urethral reconstruction similar to hypospadias repair (see Displaced Urethral Openings, p. 103).

Child/Adolescent
- ↑ ventilation of feelings regarding appearance of genitalia, rejection by peers, ability to function sexually and procreate; care for permanent urinary diversion if present.

Parents
- Support parents coping with child with a defect, multistage surgeries, possible need for permanent urinary diversion, and impact on child's future sexual functioning.
- Teach care of child: S&S of infection; clean intermittent catheterization to empty urinary reservoir.

Cryptorchidism (Cryptorchism)

- One or both testes do not descend into scrotum; risk for cancer of testes.

Signs and Symptoms
- Nonpalpable testes; affected hemiscrotum appears smaller.
- May experience infertility due to exposure of testes to body heat.

Treatment
- Orchiopexy at 6–24 months to prevent torsion.

Nursing Care
- Assess urinary functioning, I&O.
- Prevent contamination of operative site by urine and feces.
- Apply ordered cool compresses to operative site.
- Give prescribed analgesics, antibiotics.
- Teach parents to assess testes and scrotum monthly and to teach procedure to child when older.

- Abnormal location of urethral opening.
- May reflect ambiguous genitalia.

Signs and Symptoms

- **Hypospadias:** Female has opening in vagina; male has opening on lower surface of penis; penis may have downward curvature **(chordee)** due to fibrous band of tissue; penis appears hooded and crooked; small penis may appear as elongated clitoris.
- **Epispadias:** Occurs only in males; opening on dorsal surface of penis; related to defects such as exstrophy of bladder, undescended testes, short penis.

Treatment

- Circumcision delayed to preserve tissue; surgical repair.

Nursing Care

Child

Postoperative hypospadias: Assess for S&S of infection; care for indwelling catheter or stent, irrigate if ordered; avoid tub baths until stent is removed; apply prescribed antibacterial ointment to penis daily; give prescribed sedatives, analgesics, antibiotics.

Postoperative epispadias: See Exstrophy of the Bladder, Nursing Care, p. 101.

Parents

- Support coping with child with a defect, multiple surgeries, and impact on child's future sexual functioning.
- Teach S&S of infection; care of indwelling catheter such as avoid kinks in catheter, never clamp catheter, use urine-collection device in older child to promote mobility.
- Teach to encourage ↑ fluid intake.
- Teach avoidance of straddle toys, sandboxes, swimming, contact sports until permitted.

Urinary Tract Problems

Glomerulonephritis and Nephrotic Syndrome

Glomerulonephritis	Nephrotic Syndrome
• Immune-complex reaction resulting in exudative process that narrows capillaries of glomeruli. • Complication of having an infection in prior 10–14 days; organism is usually group A β-hemolytic streptococcus.	• Metabolic, biochemical, or physiochemical disturbance that occurs in glomerular capillary basement membranes causing ↓ in permeability to protein (albumin).
S&S	**S&S**
• Periorbital edema in AM; peripheral edema in PM; ↓ urine; dark-colored urine; dysuria; anorexia; pallor; irritability; lethargy; headache; ↓ BP; mild to moderate proteinuria; heart failure. • Peak incidence 6–7 yr of age.	• Periorbital edema in AM, generalized edema in PM; urine out-put; ↓ urine → anasarca; ↑ urine output; dark, frothy urine; irritability; anorexia; progressive ↓ weight; normal or ↑ BP; massive proteinuria. • Peak incidence 2–7 yr of age.
Treatment	**Treatment**
• Symptomatic recovery usually uneventful; fluid intake equal to volume of urine excreted plus insensible loss with oliguria; regular diet; ↑ K and ↑ Na with oliguria; ↑ protein with azotemia; antibiotic for persistent infection; antihypertensive for ↓ BP.	• Regular diet; ↓ Na diet with anasarca; corticosteroids; immunosuppressive if unresponsive to steroids or for relapses; occasionally diuretics and/or plasma expanders with anasarca.

Nursing Care
- Assess vital signs (VS), particularly ↑ blood pressure (BP) with glomeru-lonephritis and signs of infection with nephrotic syndrome; I&O (weigh diapers); daily weight; extent of edema; abdominal girth; urine for amount, frequency, color, clarity, odor; extent of albumin.
- Position in semi- to high-Fowler position with ↑ R or shortness of breath (SOB).
- Divide restricted fluid during waking hours; encourage intake of permitted foods; teach fluid and/or dietary restrictions.
- Protect edematous skin: Reposition every 2 hr; elevate scrotum and legs; clean and dry skin and separate skin folds with cotton clothing.
- Encourage rest until proteinuria resolves; provide appropriate age- and activity-level diversions.
- Promote a positive body image regarding physical changes related to edema and steroids.
- Teach parents about medications and their side effects; that irritability and mood swings result from disease and steroids.

Upper Gastrointestinal Tract Problems

Cleft Lip (CL) and Cleft Palate (CP)

- Congenital malformation caused by genetic aberration or teratogens such as drugs, viruses, or other toxins.
- **Cleft lip:** Unilateral or bilateral fissure in lip; more common in boys.
- **Cleft palate:** Unilateral or bilateral; complete or incomplete opening in soft and/or hard palate; may include lip; more common in girls.

Signs and Symptoms
- Difficulty feeding: ↓ ability to form vacuum with mouth; may be able to breastfeed.
- Mouth breathing with ↑ swallowed air → distended abdomen and dry mucous membranes.
- Recurrent otitis media and ↓ hearing due to inefficient eustachian tubes.
- Impaired speech due to inefficient muscles of soft palate, nasopharynx; ↓ hearing; misaligned teeth.

Treatment
- Surgical repair.
- Follow up with speech therapist, orthodontist.

Nursing Care
Preoperative
- ■ Prevent aspiration: Feed with ↑ head of bed (HOB); use CL/CP feeding device such as Haberman feeder, Pigeon bottle, Ross Gravity Flow
- ■ Burp frequently; place in partial side-lying position with ↑ HOB; gently suction oropharynx prn.

Postoperative
- ■ Prevent aspiration (see Preoperative above).
- ■ Prevent trauma to suture line by limiting crying, if possible, and maintaining position of lip-protective device; use elbow restraints if necessary; place on back or position in infant seat.
- ■ Cleanse suture line after each feeding.
- ■ Assess for ↑ swallowing that may indicate bleeding.
- ■ Give prescribed analgesic, sedative, antibiotic.

Parents
- ■ ↑ ventilation of feelings; show pictures of successful repairs; teach pre- and postoperative care; encourage cuddling to ↑ attachment.

Nasopharyngeal and Tracheoesophageal Anomalies

- ■ Congenital malformation caused by genetic aberration or teratogens such as drugs, viruses, or other toxins.
- ■ **Choanal atresia:** Lack of opening between one or both nasal passages and nasopharynx.
- ■ **Chalasia:** Incompetent cardiac sphincter.
- ■ **Esophageal atresia:** Failed esophageal development.
- ■ **Tracheoesophageal fistula:** Opening between trachea and esophagus.

Signs and Symptoms
- ■ Respiratory distress, three Cs: Coughing, Choking, Cyanosis.
- ■ Excessive salivation and drooling; abdominal distention.
- ■ During feeding: Choking, coughing, sneezing, regurgitation into mouth/nose.
- ■ Inability to pass a nasogastric tube (NGT).

Treatment
- ■ Surgical repair.

Nursing Care
Preoperative
- ■ Maintain nothing-by-mouth (NPO) status; supine with ↑ HOB; assess I&O and pulse oximetry.

- Provide ordered intravenous fluid (IVF); give prescribed antibiotics.
- Suction catheter in esophageal pouch as ordered and oropharynx as needed (PRN).

Postoperative
- Maintain airway; care for chest tubes if present; change position to prevent pneumonia; give prescribed analgesics and antibiotics.
- Give ordered gastrostomy feedings until able to tolerate oral feedings; provide mouth care; assess I&O and daily weight.
- Hold, cuddle, provide pacifier for nonnutritive sucking.

Parents
- ↑ ventilation of feelings; support attachment; encourage cuddling; discuss repair, including stay in ICU.
- Teach postop care such as suctioning, gastrostomy feedings, and skin care.

Hypertrophic Pyloric Stenosis

- Thickened muscle of pyloric sphincter narrows or obstructs opening between stomach and duodenum; presents 1–10 weeks after birth.

Signs and Symptoms
- Palpable olive-shaped mass just to right of umbilicus.
- Visible peristaltic waves across abdomen, colicky pain.
- Progressive projectile vomiting, constipation, distention of epigastrium.
- Dehydration, ↓ weight, failure to thrive.
- Metabolic alkalosis: ↑ pH, ↑ bicarbonate, ↓ Na, ↓ chloride, ↓ K.

Treatment
- Surgical repair.

Nursing Care
Preoperative
- Keep NPO; provide ordered IVF to rehydrate and electrolytes to correct imbalances.
- Maintain NGT to decompress stomach.

Postoperative
- Provide small frequent feedings of glucose, water, or electrolyte solution every 4–6 hr; then formula 24 hr later; ↑ amount and intervals between feedings gradually.

Parents
- Teach care of child; assess and support child-care skills.

Lower Gastrointestinal Problems

Colic

- Paroxysmal abdominal cramping; usually occurs >3 hr a day for >3 days a week during first 3 months.
- Multicausation theories: Immature nervous system, cow's milk allergy, ↑ fermentation and excessive swallowing of air that ↑ flatus, dietary intake of breastfeeding mother, secondhand smoke.

Signs and Symptoms

- Inconsolable, loud crying; pulls legs up to abdomen.
- Distended tense abdomen, ↑ flatus.

Treatment

- Rule out other causes for infant distress; treat symptomatically.
- No evidence-based role for medications.

Nursing Care

- Obtain history:
  - Frequency, duration, characteristics of crying; relationship of crying to time of day and feedings.
  - Infant's diet, breastfeeding mother's diet, stooling and voiding patterns.
  - Sleeping pattern, environmental stimuli.
  - Behaviors of caregivers such as methods to ↑ crying, response to crying, smoking.
- Change modifiable causes that may contribute to abdominal pain.
- **Implement 5 Ss:**
  - **S**waddle tightly in receiving blanket.
  - **S**ucking: Encourage pacifier, mother's nipple.
  - **S**ide or **S**tomach lying while monitored.
  - **S**hushing sounds: Use white noise machine or CD tape.
  - **S**winging: Provide rhythmic movements with bed vibrator, swing, or hammock.
- Teach feeding techniques: Proper placement of breast or nipple; give small, frequent, feedings slowly; burp often; use bottles that ↑ air swallowing; provide calm environment.
- Apply pressure to abdomen with hand; massage abdomen.
- Eliminate secondhand smoke.
- Encourage parents to seek respite from child care.

Obstructions: Volvulus and Intussusception

- **Intussusception:** Proximal segment of bowel telescopes into a distal segment; often at ileocecal valve; presents at 3–12 months; requires nonsurgical hydrostatic reduction or surgical repair.
- **Volvulus:** Intestine twists around itself; presents during first 6 months; linked to malrotation of intestine; requires surgical repair.

Signs and Symptoms
- Intussusception triad:
  - Acute onset of severe paroxysmal abdominal pain.
  - Palpable sausage-shaped mass.
  - Currant-jelly stools.
- Inconsolable crying, kicking, drawing legs up to abdomen, grunting respirations due to abdominal distention, vomiting, lethargy.
- Untreated: Necrosis, perforation, peritonitis, and sepsis.

Treatment
- Surgical repair of both conditions; hydrostatic reduction for intussusception.

Nursing Care
Preprocedure/Surgery
- Maintain NPO and gastric decompression; give ordered IVF and electrolytes.
- Give prescribed analgesics, antibiotics.

Postprocedure/Surgery
- Give ordered IVF and electrolytes.
- Assess VS; amount and characteristics of stool.
- Assess passage of contrast material if hydrostatic reduction used for intussusception.
- Give ordered oral feedings; encourage breastfeeding to ↓ infant constipation.
- Encourage parental visits to ↓ separation anxiety in older infant.

Intestinal Malformations

	Imperforate Anus	Megacolon (Hirschsprung)
	Stricture or absence of anus with simple to complex genitourinary and pelvic organ involvement.	Lack of parasympathetic ganglion cells in portion of bowel leads to bowel enlargement proximal to defect.
S&S	**S&S**	**S&S**
	• Failure to pass meconium stool, abdominal distention. • Meconium on perineum; meconium in vagina or in urine due to a fistula.	• Neonate: Abdominal distention, vomiting, failure to pass meconium within 48 hr of birth, enterocolitis. • Infant/child: Occurs gradually; pellet- or ribbon-like, foul-smelling stool; refusal of food; abdominal distention; chronic constipation; S&S of intestinal obstruction.
Treatment	**Treatment**	**Treatment**
	• Surgical repair depends on extent of anomaly; repair with possible temporary colostomy.	• Resection with temporary colostomy, stool softeners, dietary modifications.

Nursing Care

Preoperative

- Maintain NPO; administer ordered IVF, electrolytes; assess I&O.
- Implement and maintain ordered gastric decompression.
- Give prescribed analgesics, antibiotics.
- Assist with diagnostic tests to identify related anomalies.

Postoperative

- **Assess VS;** amount and characteristics of stool; give IVF, electrolytes.
- **Extent of surgery dictates care:** Provide ordered anal dilations; care for temporary colostomy; implement bowel management program; give ordered oral feedings; encourage breastfeeding because it ↑ infant constipation.

Parents

- Promote attachment with neonate.
- Encourage visits to ↓ separation anxiety in older infant.

Diabetes Mellitus (DM) in Children

- Disorder of carbohydrate (CHO), protein, and fat metabolism causing hyperglycemia that ultimately precipitates multiorgan complications; for more detail, including information about hyperglycemia, hypoglycemia, DKA, HHNS, Somogyi effect, and dawn phenomenon, see Tab 6 MEDSURG, Diabetes Mellitus, p. 191, and Alterations in Blood Glucose Associated With DM, p. 192.
- **Type 1:** Hereditary and environment; 60% of genetic susceptibility related to human leukocyte antigen (HLA); HLA ↑ susceptibility to a trigger such as viruses, cow's milk, or chemical irritants that initiate an autoimmune process that destroys beta cells.
- **Type 2:** ↓ release of insulin and/or insulin secretion is inhibited or inactivated; increasing incidence in school-age children and adolescents; more common with obesity, inactivity, ↑ fat and ↑ calorie diets, and in Native Americans.

Signs and Symptoms
- Type 1: Onset is rapid and obvious, three Ps (<u>P</u>olyuria, <u>P</u>olyphagia, <u>P</u>olydipsia), enuresis, fatigue.
- Type 2: Onset is gradual, fatigue, obesity, recurrent UTIs and vaginal infections.

Treatment
- Dietary and lifestyle changes and medications to maintain normal glucose levels (see Tab 6 MEDSURG, Alterations in Blood Glucose Associated With DM, p. 192; Tab 7 MEDS, Hypoglycemics, p. 264; and Insulin, p. 265).

Nursing Care
- Design strategies appropriate for developmental and cognitive level; use pictures and play; be interactive.
- See Tab 6 MEDSURG, Alterations in Blood Glucose Associated With DM, p. 192; Tab 7 MEDS, Hypoglycemics—Nursing Implications, p. 264; and Insulin—Nursing Care, p. 264.
- **Preschoolers:** Teach about DM and food choices on child's cognitive level.
- **School-age children:** Teach self-monitoring of blood glucose (SMBG), urine testing, and insulin injection such as syringe-loaded injector (Inject-Ease) or self-contained device (NovoPen); S&S of complications.
- **Adolescents:** Explore need for conformity with peers and nonadherence with medical regimen; ↑ self-care; ↑ motivation with day off or occasional dietary treat.
- **Self-injection of insulin:** Inject same area for six to eight injections or up to 1 month; abdomen and thigh best; use shortest, smallest-gauge needle possible and pinch technique; insert needle at 90°; track injection sites.

- **Nutrition:** Teach glycemic index of foods, appropriate snacks, sugar substitutes with moderation; support personal and cultural preferences.
- **Exercise:** Encourage daily exercise; additional food intake ½ hr before activity and then every 45 min to 1 hr throughout.
- **Continued supervision**: Promote multidisciplinary approach; refer to American Diabetes Association.

Congenital Heart Defects

Defects With Increased Pulmonary Blood Flow

Ventricular Septal Defect
- Abnormal opening between ventricles; ↑ right ventricular pressure causing pulmonary hypertension and right ventricular hypertrophy.
- S&S: Low harsh murmur throughout systole.

Atrial Septal Defect
- Abnormal opening between atria; right atrial and ventricular enlargement stretches conduction fibers, causing dysrhythmias.
- S&S: Murmur heard high in chest with fixed splitting of second heart sound.

Patent Ductus Arteriosus
- Patency of fetal connection between aorta and pulmonary artery; ↑ left atrial and ventricular workload causing↑ pulmonary vascular congestion.
- S&S: May be asymptomatic; machinery-type murmur throughout heartbeat in left second or third intercostal space; bounding pulse; widened pulse pressure.

Defects With Decreased Pulmonary Blood Flow

Tetralogy of Fallot
- Four defects: Pulmonary valve stenosis, ventricular septal defect, overriding aorta, right ventricular hypertrophy.
- S&S: Depends on extent of defects; mild to acute cyanosis; murmur; acute episodes of cyanosis and hypoxia (**blue spells, tet spells**) when energy demands exceed oxygen supply such as when crying or feeding.

Tricuspid Atresia
- Absence of tricuspid valve; no communication from right atrium to right ventricle; death occurs without connection between right and left sides of heart such as patent foramen ovale, atrial septal defect, patent ductus arteriosus, ventricular septal defect.
- S&S: Cyanosis, tachycardia, dyspnea.

Defects With Mixed Blood Flow

Transposition of the Great Vessels
- Aorta exits from right ventricle and pulmonary artery exits from left ventricle; no communication between pulmonary and systemic circulation; death occurs without connection between right and left sides of heart such as patent foramen ovale, atrial septal defect, patent ductus arteriosus, ventricular septal defect.
- S&S: Mild to severe cyanosis; heart sounds and other S&S depend on associated defects.

Truncus Arteriosus
- Blood from both ventricles enters single great vessel that arises from base of heart directing blood to both pulmonary and systemic circulation; more blood flows to pulmonary arteries because of ↓ resistance than systemic circulation, causing hypoxia.
- S&S: Systolic murmur, single semilunar valve produces loud second heart sound that is not split, variable cyanosis, delayed growth, activity intolerance.

Obstructive Defects

Coarctation of the Aorta
- Narrowing of aorta near insertion of ductus arteriosus causing ↑ pressure proximal to defect and ↓ pressure distal to defect; ↓ blood flow out of ventricles.
- S&S: ↑ BP; bounding radial and carotid pulses; lower extremities have ↓ BP, weak or absent femoral pulses, cool to touch.

Pulmonic Stenosis
- Narrowing of pulmonary valve; resistance to blood flow causing ↓ pulmonary blood flow and right ventricular hypertrophy.
- S&S: Murmur, mild cyanosis, cardiomegaly, or may be asymptomatic.

Aortic Stenosis
- Narrowing of aortic valve; resistance to blood flow, causing ↓ cardiac output; left ventricular hypertrophy; ↑ pulmonary vascular congestion.
- S&S: Murmur, faint pulses, ↓ BP, tachycardia, poor feeding, exercise intolerance.

Complications of Congenital Heart Defects

Heart Failure (HF)

- Heart unable to pump blood to meet body's metabolic demands due to ↓ myocardial contractility and ↑ volume of blood returning to heart (**preload**) ↑ resistance against blood being ejected from left ventricle (**afterload**).
- S&S: Pulse; weak peripheral pulses; ↑ BP; gallop rhythm; diaphoresis; ↓ urinary output; pale, cool extremities; fatigue; restlessness; weakness; anorexia.

Pulmonary Congestion

- Excessive amount of blood in pulmonary vascular bed; fluid moves into interstitial spaces when pulmonary capillary pressure exceeds plasma osmotic pressure (pulmonary edema); associated with left-sided HF.
- S&S: ↑ Pulse, dyspnea, retractions in infants, flaring nares, wheezing, grunting, cyanosis, cough, hoarseness, orthopnea, activity intolerance.

Systemic Venous Congestion

- ↑ pressure and pooling of blood in venous circulation.
- Called cor pulmonale when due to primary lung disease such as cystic fibrosis.
- S&S: ↑ weight, peripheral and periorbital edema, hepatomegaly, ascites, distended neck veins.

Nursing Care of Children With Congenital Heart Defects

Child

- Assess for S&S specific to defect, hypoxia, pulmonary congestion, systemic venous congestion, HF.
- Assess:
  - VS, heart and breath sounds, pulse oximetry, ECG.
  - I&O, daily weight, maintain ordered fluid restriction.
  - Electrolyte imbalances, especially hypokalemia (↓ BP, ↑ P, irritability, drowsiness) → ↑ risk of digoxin toxicity.
- Facilitate breathing: ↑ HOB 30°–45°; avoid constipation and constrictive clothing; provide ordered oxygen.
- Manage hypercyanotic spells (tet spell): Interrupt activity; soothe if crying; hold in knee chest position with head ↑ to limit venous return to heart.
- Provide ordered small feedings or gavage (usually every 2–3 hr); use soft nipple with large hole to ↓ work of sucking; burp frequently.
- Provide age-appropriate teaching to prepare child for surgery.

Parents

- Support grieving; discuss specifics of disorder and appropriate care.
- Teach to treat child and siblings equally to ↓ over dependency; set age-appropriate goals within child's activity tolerance; provide consistent discipline to ↓ secondary gains.
- Encourage delegation to prevent parental exhaustion.

Respiratory Problems

Respiratory Tract Infections (RTIs)

- **Nasopharyngitis (common cold):** Inflammation of nasopharynx.
- **Streptococcal pharyngitis:** Group A β-hemolytic streptococcus (GABHS) infects upper airway; can lead to acute rheumatic fever or acute glomerulonephritis.
- **Tonsillitis:** Inflammation of lymphatic tissue of pharynx particularly palatine tonsils.
- **Influenza:** Influenza virus type A or B causes inflammation of respiratory tract.
- **Otitis media:** Acute infection of middle ear usually due to *Streptococcus pneumoniae* or *Haemophilus influenzae*.
- **Bronchiolitis:** Bronchiolar inflammation usually due to respiratory syncytial virus (RSV).
- **Pneumonia:** Inflammation of pulmonary parenchyma.
- **Epiglottitis:** Inflammation of epiglottis.
- **Laryngitis:** Inflammation of larynx.
- **Laryngotracheobronchitis:** Inflammation of larynx, trachea, bronchi; causative organism identified via C&S; rapid immunofluorescent antibody (IFA) or enzyme-linked immunosorbent assay (ELISA) techniques for RSV detection.

Factors Influencing Occurrence of RTIs

- **Age of child:** <3 months protected by maternal antibodies; infant and toddler have ↑ incidence of viral infections; school-age have ↑ incidence of pneumonia and β-hemolytic streptococcus infections.
- **Size of child:** Infants and toddlers have small diameter airways and short, open eustachian tubes, increasing risk of otitis media.
- **Season:** Viral infections particularly respiratory syncytial virus in winter and spring; asthmatic bronchitis in winter.
- **Living conditions**: Secondhand smoke, day-care centers, multiple siblings, crowded conditions.

- **Preexisting medical condition:** Immune deficiencies; malnutrition; allergies; medical problems such as cystic fibrosis, Down syndrome, and asthma.

Common Signs and Symptoms

- Irritability, restlessness, anorexia, malaise, chills, muscular aches, headache.
- Irritation of pharynx and nasal passages, nasal discharge, mouth or breath odor.
- ↑ VS, cough, dyspnea, cervical lymphadenopathy.
- Seizures may occur with T > 102°F.

Specific Signs and Symptoms

- *Laryngitis:* Hoarseness.
- *Tonsillitis:* Tonsils covered with exudates.
- *Epiglottitis:* Large cherry-red edematous epiglottis; slow, quiet breathing; agitation; drooling; sore throat; no spontaneous cough.
- *Otitis media:* Pulling at ears or rolling head side to side; earache; sucking or chewing ↑ pain; bulging red eardrum; may exhibit hearing loss, vomiting, diarrhea.
- *Laryngotracheobronchitis (croup):*
  - *Stage I:* Fear, hoarseness, barking cough, inspiratory stridor.
  - *Stage II:* Dyspnea, retractions, use of accessory muscles.
  - *Stage III:* Restlessness, pallor, diaphoresis, ↑ R, S&S of hypoxia, CO_2 retention.
  - *Stage IV:* Cyanosis, cessation of breathing.

Commonalities of Treatment

- Promote respirations: ↑ humidity with mist tent, humidifier, steam from hot shower in closed bathroom, or saline nasal spray; bronchodilators; ↑ HOB; oxygen; oropharyngeal suctioning except with croup syndromes.
- ↑ temp: Give antipyretics but avoid aspirin to prevent Reye syndrome; cool liquids, chest physical therapy (PT) to ↑ expectoration.
- ↑ hydration: Oral rehydration such as Pedialyte or Infalyte; sports drinks such as Gatorade and Exceed; high-calorie liquids; provide IVF if unable to drink.
- ↓ rest; BR or quiet activity.
- ↑ comfort: Analgesics, heat, cold, gargles, or troches for sore throat, cough suppressants for dry cough.

Treatment for Specific RTIs

- *Bacterial infections:* Judicious use of antibiotics such as amoxicillin, second-generation cephalosporins or erythromycin; rifampin may be added for GABHS.
- *Tonsillitis:* Surgical removal of tonsils and adenoids that obstruct breathing or for recurrent infections.

- *Otitis media:* Antibiotic eardrops, local heat, myringotomy for persistent effusion or hearing loss.
- *Epiglottis:* Corticosteroids, endotracheal intubation or tracheostomy for severe respiratory distress.
- *Croup:* Corticosteroids, nebulized epinephrine.
- *Respiratory syncytial virus:* Ribavirin (Virazole).

Nursing Care

- **Acute care:**
  - Institute and maintain droplet precautions.
  - Assess risk for respiratory obstruction.
  - Collect sputum cultures before beginning antibiotics (best in a.m.).
  - Support parents and child with frightening SOB or airway obstruction.
  - Keep upright (sit on lap), supine, or side-lying position with neck slightly extended (**sniff position**).
  - Provide ordered humidified oxygen; assess pulse oximetry.
  - ↑ fluids to replace loss from fever, perspiration, ↑ respirations, and to liquefy secretions.
  - Manage secretions (nasal aspirator, oropharyngeal suctioning except with croup syndromes); chest PT.
  - Give prescribed antibiotics, decongestants, analgesics.
  - Maintain BR, calm environment; engage in age-appropriate quiet diversionary activities.
- **Teach preventive measures:** Frequent hand hygiene; containment of soiled tissues; cough or sneeze into tissue or elbow; avoid sharing eating utensils, glasses, or towels; formula-feeding of infants in upright position to ↓ fluid entering eustachian tubes.
- **Postoperative T&A:** Maintain side-lying position with HOB ↑ 30°; discourage coughing, throat clearing, nose blowing; apply ice collar; offer ice chips, ice pops, diluted juice; avoid dairy products or red-colored fluids; give prescribed analgesics to promote comfort; assess for frequent swallowing that may indicate bleeding.
- **Postoperative myringotomy:** Place on affected side to ↑ ear drainage; apply ordered heat or cold; clean and apply moisture barrier to pinna to protect skin from drainage; recognize S&S of ↓ hearing; teach parents to prevent bath and shampoo water from entering ear; feed in upright position; eliminate allergens; encourage follow-up care.

Asthma

- Stimulus causes inflammation that ↑ mucus, mucosal edema, bronchospasm; this traps air in lungs → chronic tissue irritation, scarring, hyperinflation.
- Peak expiratory flow rate: ↓ maximum flow of air forcefully exhaled in 1 min.

- Occurs due to allergens such as mold, pollen, dust mites, and cockroach allergen or nonimmunological stimuli such as infections, exercise, cold air, odors, smoke, stress, and dairy products.
- Characterized by remissions and exacerbations; may be mild and intermittent to severe, persistent, intractable (status asthmaticus).

Signs and Symptoms

- Dyspnea, dry cough, prolonged expirations with wheezing, sternal retractions, flaring nares, barrel chest.
- Prodromal exacerbation: Rhinorrhea; low-grade fever; itching on neck, chest, and upper back; anorexia; headache; irritability; restlessness; fatigue; chest tightness; anxiety.
- Progression of exacerbation: Frothy, clear, gelatinous sputum; productive cough; ↑ R; SOB; pale face with red ears; lips dark red progressing to cyanosis; tripod or orthopneic position; hyperresonance on chest percussion; breath sounds coarse with sonorous crackles.
- Imminent ventilatory failure: SOB with absence of breath sounds.

Treatment

- Removal of stimulus.
- Long-term control medications (**preventer medications**): Oral or inhaled corticosteroids; NSAIDs to ↓ inflammation and allergic response.
- Quick-relief medications (**rescue medications**): ↓ exacerbations;
β-adrenergics and anticholinergics ↑ bronchodilation.
- Emergency protocol: Three treatments with short-acting β-adrenergic spaced at 20–30 min; systemic prednisone; and an anticholinergic; hydration with caution to prevent pulmonary edema; oxygen with caution to prevent CO_2 narcosis.

Nursing Care

- Support child and parent in coping with chronic illness and fear due to SOB.
- Prevent exacerbations: Avoid triggers such as dairy products and animals; allergy-proof home such as eliminate carpets, drapes, down bedding; wet-mop floors; assess status via peak expiratory flowmeter (PEFM).
- Care during exacerbation: Provide calm presence; assess cardiopulmonary status; place in ↑ Fowler position; encourage pursed-lip breathing; give prescribed medications.
- Teach how to use a PEFM
  - Measures respiratory volume of one forced expiration; begin with indicator at bottom of scale; stand straight, take a deep breath, place

mouthpiece in mouth, blow out as hard and fast as possible; note result on scale.
- Repeat 3 times and record highest value.
  Green: Under control.
  Yellow: Exacerbation; may indicate need to ↑ maintenance dose of medications.
  Red: Severe airway narrowing; give rescue medication.

Cystic Fibrosis (CF)

- Causes ↑ viscosity of mucus from exocrine glands and abnormal glandular secretion of ions. It is an autosomal recessive disease.

Effects on Organ Systems
Respiratory System
- Mucus obstructs respiratory passages → ↓ expectoration and ↓ gas exchange.
- Mucus stagnation causes hypercapnia; hypoxia; acidosis; infection.
- ↑ lung dysfunction → atelectasis, emphysema, cor pulmonale, respiratory failure, and death.

Pancreas
- ↓ secretion of chloride and bicarbonate.
- Mucus blocks enzymes from reaching duodenum, causing ↓ digestion of fats, proteins, and CHO; fibrosis may result in DM.

Liver
- Local biliary obstruction; fibrosis causes biliary cirrhosis.

Reproductive System
- Delayed puberty; females may be infertile; males usually sterile due to mucus blocking sperm.

Integumentary system
- ↑ Secretion of sodium and chloride in saliva and sweat; hyperthermic conditions cause hyponatremic alkalosis, hypochloremia, and dehydration.

Signs and Symptoms
- Variable; may be asymptomatic for months or yr.
- Suspected with meconium ileus, failure to regain weight loss at birth, and failure to thrive.
- Frequent RTIs, nonproductive cough, wheezing.
- Chest x-ray shows atelectasis and emphysema; pulmonary function tests reveal small airway dysfunction.

- Foul-smelling, pale, bulky, watery stools (**steatorhea**): stools contain ↑ fat and pancreatic enzymes.
- Positive sweat chloride test: Chlorine concentration >60 mEq/L.
- Chronic S&S: ↓ salivation, paroxysmal cough, dyspnea, cyanosis, barrel chest, distended abdomen, thin extremities, clubbing of fingers and toes, rectal prolapse, F&E imbalances, bruising due to↓ vitamin K.

Treatment

- Oral fluids and mucolytic enzymes to ↑ mucus viscosity; chest PT.
- Bronchodilators, anti-inflammatories, antibiotics.
- ↑ protein and ↑ calorie diet; salt supplements prn; pancreatic enzymes with meals and snacks to ↓ steatorrhea and ↑ growth; vitamins A, D, E, and K.
- Daily aerobic exercise.
- Lung transplant.

Nursing Care

Child

Respiratory functioning

- Assess lung sounds; S&S of respiratory distress.
- Balance rest and activity; ↑ fluids to ↑ mucus viscosity.
- Teach how to ↑ expectoration such as huffing on expectoration and use of flutter mucus clearance device.

GI Functioning

- Assess weight, abdominal distention, and stools for characteristics and frequency.
- Assess for S&S of intestinal obstruction.
- Teach to ↑ protein and ↑ calories; give pancreatic enzymes with food.
- Ensure adequate salt intake, particularly in hot weather.
- Use perianal skin barrier to protect skin from GI enzymes.

Psychosocial support

- Provide age-appropriate support to ↑ coping with chronic illness, respiratory equipment, invasive procedures, and infertility.
- Promote a positive self-image.

Parents

- Assist parents with shock and guilt (each contributed a gene), chronicity of illness, and potential for death.
- Teach chest PT such as postural drainage, percussion, and vibration; perform daily in AM and PM and between meals to prevent vomiting.
- Teach about ThAIRapy vest to provide chest wall oscillation.
- Teach diaphragmatic breathing and coughing.
- Encourage child's independence and limit overindulgence to ↑ secondary gains.
- Ensure routine immunizations; flu vaccine at 6 months and then yearly.
- Refer for genetic counseling and to Cystic Fibrosis Foundation.

Disseminated Intravascular Coagulation (DIC)

- Secondary disorder of coagulation that complicates a primary pathological process such as hypoxia, acidosis, shock, burns, sepsis, and necrotizing enterocolitis.
- Laboratory results indicate prolonged prothrombin time (PT), partial thromboplastin time (PTT), and thrombin time (TT); ↓ platelet count, ↓ fibrinogen; fragmented red blood cells (RBCs).
- Has two concurrent phases:
  - **Phase 1:** Abnormal stimulation of coagulation process ↑ thrombin beyond what can be neutralized; this leads to conversion of fibrinogen to fibrin, causing aggregation and destruction of platelets promoting thrombi that impede blood flow with eventual tissue necrosis.
  - **Phase 2:** Fibrinolytic mechanism is activated → ↑ destruction of clotting factors → uncontrolled hemorrhage.

Signs and Symptoms
- Petechiae, purpura, bleeding from break in skin such as from a venipuncture or surgical site, ↓ BP.
  - Organ dysfunction related to infarction and ischemia.

Treatment
- Control of underlying cause.
- Platelets, fresh-frozen plasma, exchange transfusions with fresh blood.
- IV heparin when not responding to previous therapy.

Nursing Care
Child
- Depends on extent of bleeding, thrombus formation, and organs involved; child usually is in PICU.
- Administer prescribed IV infusions, blood transfusions, and heparin therapy.

Parents
- Support coping with critically ill child.

Hemophilia

- X-linked recessive genetic disorder; possible gene mutation.
- Males usually are affected and females are carriers.
- **Hemophilia A (classic hemophilia):** Associated with deficiency of factor VIII.
- **Hemophilia B (Christmas disease):** Associated with deficiency of factor IX.

- Lack of a blood-clotting factor affects coagulation cascade, prolonging clot formation and bleeding.
- Prenatal testing identifies affected fetus.
- Tests distinguish specific factor deficiencies: PT; PTT; thromboplastin generation test (TGT); whole blood clotting time; prothrombin consumption test; fibrinogen level.

Signs and Symptoms

- Bleeding
- Into joints (**hemarthrosis**): Joint stiffness, tingling, ache; followed by warmth, redness, swelling, pain, loss of movement, joint deformities, and impaired growth.
  - Into brain: Headache, slurred speech, ↑ LOC.
  - Into subcutaneous and intramuscular tissue: Ecchymosis, red spots (**petechiae**)
  - Into GI tract: Black tarry stools, abdominal pain.
  - From nose (**epistaxis**).

Treatment

- Replacement of missing clotting factor.
- Analgesics to ↓ pain; **RICE** protocol: Rest, Ice, Compression, Elevation.
- Corticosteroids and nonsteroidal anti-inflammatories for hemarthrosis and inflammation of synovial membranes (**synovitis**).
- PT; weight control to ↓ stress on joints.

Nursing Care

Child

- Identify bleeding event; provide factor replacement.
- Rest joints; ROM after acute episode subsides.
- Prevent bleeding; Teach to use soft toothbrush, water pick, and electric razor; avoid contact sports.
- Encourage to wear medical alert identification.
- Teach to disclose condition before invasive procedures.
- Support child and adolescent in learning self-care.
- Explore coping with chronic disease, vocational, financial, and childbearing issues.

Parents

- Encourage ventilation of feelings about child with chronic illness, particularly the mother because it is X-linked; refer for genetic counseling.
- Safety-proof house and toys; supervise activity.
- Discuss need for multidisciplinary follow-up.

Anemia

Iron Deficiency	Sickle Cell	β-Thalassemia
• Inadequate amount of iron to make hemoglobin (Hb), a component of RBCs, which causes anemia. • Caused by ↓ dietary iron; infant has iron reserve for only 5–6 months. • Children receiving only milk have no source of dietary iron **(milk babies)**.	• Autosomal recessive disorder: Homozygous patient will develop sickle cell anemia; heterozygous patient will be a carrier. • More common in African Americans. • HbS forms long, slender crystals causing sickle-shaped RBCs, ↓ RBCs, Hb <9 g/dL; precipitated by dehydration; acidosis; ↑T; hypoxia. • Cloudy mixture with sickle-turbidity test (Sickledex) for newborn screening. • Hb electrophoresis to determine if patient is heterozygous or homozygous. • Complications: Problems with bones and joints, CNS, spleen, eyes, liver, reproductive system, kidneys, and lungs (chest syndrome: Pulmonary infiltrate → chest pain, ↑T, ↑ R, cough, wheezing, hypoxia).	• Autosomal recessive disorder more common in people of Mediterranean descent. • ↓ synthesis of β-chain polypeptides → ↓ globin molecules. • Inability to maintain erythropoiesis commensurate with hemolysis; RBC changes, ↓ Hct, ↓ Hb, ↑ HbF, ↑ HbgA$_2$. • **Thalassemia major (Cooley anemia)** homozygous form that results in death without transfusions.

Continued

Iron Deficiency	Sickle Cell	β-Thalassemia
S&S	**S&S**	**S&S**
• Slow onset. • ↑ P, pallor, ↓ motor development, weakness, dizziness. • ↓ RBC, ↓ Hb, ↓ Hct, ↑ total iron-binding capacity, ↓ serum-iron concentration.	• Longer than 6 months; failure to thrive; ↑ risk of infection. **Vaso-occlusive crisis** • Pain episode: Sickled cells obstruct blood vessels, causing occlusion, ischemia, and necrosis; pain and swelling of hands and feet; abdominal pain; arthralgia; ↑ T; prolonged penile erection **(priapism).** **Sequestration crisis** • Pooling of blood → splenomegaly; hepatomegaly; ↓ BP; lethargy; hypovolemia; shock. **Aplastic crisis** • Profound anemia due to ↓ RBC production and ↑ RBC destruction; lethargy; SOB; altered mental status; and S&S of heart failure. **Hyperhemolytic crisis** • ↑ RBC destruction → jaundice, reticulocytosis; suggests coexisting disorders.	• Fatigue, anorexia, ↑ T. • Bronze, freckled skin. • Splenomegaly, hepatomegaly. • Thickened cranial bones, malocclusion of jaw, chipmunklike facies, ↓ bone growth, bone pain. • Delayed sexual maturation.

Iron Deficiency	Sickle Cell	β-Thalassemia
Treatment	**Treatment to prevent sickling**	**Treatment**
• Breast milk or 1 L/day of iron-fortified formula for first 12 months. • Ferrous sulfate supplement may cause gastric irritation and greenish/black stools.	• Oxygen, ↑ fluids, maintain electrolyte and acid-base balance, hydroxyurea, erythropoietin. **Treatment during crisis** • BR to ↓ oxygen demands, rest joints, give analgesics, ↑ fluids, correct electrolytes, treat acidosis. • Blood transfusions or exchange transfusions to replace sickle cells; antibiotics; oxygen if SOB; oxygen will not reverse sickling. • Chelation therapy to ↓ iron overload.	• Blood transfusions (may be every 3 weeks); vitamin C ↑ iron excretion; chelation therapy. • Splenectomy if splenomegaly interferes with breathing or if RBC destruction is extreme. • Bone marrow transplant.
Nursing Care	**Nursing Care**	**Nursing Care**
• Assess for S&S; give iron-fortified milk and cereals or breast milk. • Give iron via a straw to ↓ staining teeth and with orange juice between meals to ↑ absorption. • Balance activity and rest.	• Assess for S&S; implement interventions to prevent hypoxia; dehydration; acidosis; and ↑ temp, which precipitates sickling. **During crises** • Give prescribed medications such as analgesics, antipyretics, and electrolytes; give ordered IVF and blood transfusions; maintain BR with ↑ HOB; support joints on pillows and when moving.	• Support coping with transfusions and chelation therapy. • Arrange therapy around lifestyle. • Support adolescents with potential infertility. • Teach that screening fetus for β-thalassemia is available.

Cancer

Leukemia

- Unrestricted proliferation of immature white blood cells (WBCs) in blood-forming tissues.
- Leukocyte count is low and immature cells (**blasts**) are high.
- Blast cells compete for and deprive normal cells of nutrients essential for metabolism, causing anemia from ↑ RBCs, infection from ↑ neutrophils, bleeding from ↓ platelets.
- Leukemic cells may infiltrate other organs such as spleen, liver, lymph nodes, and CNS.

Classification

- Acute lymphoid leukemia (ALL) and acute myelogenous leukemia (AML).
- Each have subtypes that have therapeutic and prognostic implications.

Signs and Symptoms

- Pallor, fatigue, irritability; ↑T, anorexia; ↓ weight.
- Bleeding tendencies: bruising, bleeding from mucous membranes, petechiae, hemorrhage.
- Bone and joint pain; enlarged liver, spleen, lymph nodes; CNS involvement.
- Usually occurs 2–6-yr-old child; onset is insidious to acute.

Treatment

- Based on staging.
- IV and intrathecal chemotherapy given via four-phase protocol to achieve remission, ↓ tumor burden, ↑ CNS involvement, and preserve remission.
- Bone marrow transplant.

Nursing Care for Child With SCA or β-Thalassemia

- Support parents and child coping with a genetic, chronic illness and potential for death during crises.
- Refer for genetic counseling and continued medical care.
- Prevent infection: Give flu and pneumococcal vaccines; avoid sources of infection.
- Balance activity and rest.
- Teach to avoid contact sports to prevent splenic rupture.
- Support child and adolescent coping with multiple transfusions, delayed sexual maturation, and body-image issues.
- Teach child about disorder and refer to supportive organizations such as Cooley's Anemia Foundation.

Nursing Care

■ Interventions depend on side effects of medication regimen, extent of myelosuppression, degree of leukemic infiltration.
■ Handle gently to ↓ pain, bleeding, fractures.
■ Emotional support for child and parents coping with diagnosis of cancer; invasive tests; chronic course; potential for relapse, death.
■ Assess VS especially T and BP; balance rest and quiet play.
■ Teach infection prevention such as hand hygiene, avoid crowds, and people with an infection.
■ Support child coping with side effects of antineoplastic therapies (see Tab 6, MEDSURG, Care of Patients With Cancer, p. 176).
■ Give prescribed chemotherapeutic and analgesic medications.

Wilms Tumor (Nephroblastoma)

■ Malignant tumor of kidney; possibly genetic; usually occurs < age 5 yr.
■ Associated with congenital disorders such as genitourinary problems.
■ Tumor compresses body tissues, causing secondary metabolic problems.
■ May be encapsulated for long period; metastasizes to lung, liver, bone, and brain.

Classification

■ Stages I to V, depending on confinement to kidney, extent of metastasis, if tumor is bilateral.

Signs and Symptoms

■ Presents as nontender, firm mass deep within unilateral flank.
■ Fatigue; ↓ weight; malaise; ↑ temp; hematuria and ↑ BP may occur.
■ Clinical indicators of lung metastasis: Dyspnea, cough, SOB, chest pain.

Treatment

■ Radiation or/and chemotherapy before and/or after surgery.
■ Excision of adrenal gland, affected regional lymph nodes, adjacent organs.
■ One kidney excised if unilateral; one kidney excised and partial nephrectomy of less affected kidney if bilateral.

Nursing Care

■ Depends on side effects of medication regimen and extent of myelosuppression.
■ Ensure that all primary health-care providers know not to palpate abdomen to prevent dissemination of cancer cells or rupture of tumor capsule.
■ Assess VS, particularly temp and BP.
■ Teach infection prevention such as hand hygiene, and avoid crowds and people with an infection; provide balance between rest and quiet play.

■ Give prescribed chemotherapeutic, analgesic medications.
■ Teach turning, coughing, deep breathing to prevent respiratory problems because operative site is close to diaphragm.
■ Provide emotional support for child and parents coping with diagnosis of cancer, invasive tests, chronic course, potential for relapse and death.
■ Support child who is coping with side effects of antineoplastic therapies (see Tab 6, MEDSURG, Care of Patients With Cancer, p. 176).

Neurological Problems

Neural Tube Defects

Spina Bifida Occulta
■ Defect of vertebrae with intact spinal cord and meninges.

Signs and Symptoms
■ May not be visible or may have superficial signs in lumbosacral area such as tufts of hair, angiomatous nevi, dimple, subcutaneous lipomas.
■ Progressive disturbance of gait; ↓ bowel and bladder control.

Spina Bifida Cystica
■ Saclike protrusion on back.
■ Two most common types:
  ■ **Meningocele:** Exposed sac contains meninges and spinal fluid.
  ■ **Myelomeningocele (meningomyelocele):** Sac contains spinal cord, nerve roots, spinal fluid, meninges. Myelomeningocele is associated with other malformations such as intestinal, cardiac, renal, urinary, and orthopedic.

Signs and Symptoms
■ Vary, depending on anatomical level and extent of defect; sensory disturbances parallel motor impairments.
■ Joint deformities due to denervation to ↓ extremities and flexion and extension contractures; talipes valgus or varus contractures; kyphosis; lumbosacral scoliosis; hip dislocation.
■ **Defect below second lumbar vertebra:** Flaccid, partial paralysis of legs; varying degrees of ↓ sensation; continuous dribbling of urine and overflow incontinence; no bowel control and possible rectal prolapse.
■ **Defect below third sacral vertebra:** No motor impairment; ↓ bowel and bladder control.

Treatment
■ Surgery within 24–72 hr to ↓ stretching of nerve roots and ↓ risk for trauma to sac, hydrocephalus, infection.
■ Eventually artificial sphincters and reservoirs may be created surgically.

Nursing Care
Infant Preoperative
- Keep naked in radiant warmer to prevent trauma to sac.
- Keep prone even when feeding.

Infant Postoperative
- Place in prone or partial side-lying position.
- Use sterile, moist, nonadherent dressing to site to ↓ drying; change every 2–4 hr.
- Assess for S&S of infection such as fever, irritability, lethargy, nuchal rigidity.
- Assess for leaks, tears, abrasions, hydrocephalus, ↑ ICP.
- Keep area free of urine and feces.
- Use Credé maneuver to empty bladder or ordered straight catheterization.
- Keep hips in slight abduction; perform ordered PROM to knees, ankles, and feet; for older child, use ordered braces, walking devices, and wheelchair.

Child
- Teach clean intermittent catheterization. Incontinence is most stressful for child's social development.

Parents
- Support coping with decision to abort if identified in utero, lifelong care of infant with multiple neurological, genitourinary, and musculoskeletal problems.
- Involve in care; refer to Spina Bifida Association of America.

Hydrocephalus

- Abnormal ↑ cerebrospinal fluid (CSF) in ventricular system.

Communicating Hydrocephalus
- ↓ absorption of CSF within subarachnoid space.
- Often due to infection, trauma, thick arachnoid membrane or meninges.

Noncommunicating Hydrocephalus
- Obstruction of flow of CSF through ventricular system.
- Usually due to neoplasm, hematoma, or congenital herniation of medulla through foramen magnum.

Signs and Symptoms
- ↑ head size in infant is due to open sutures and bulging fontanels.
- Sclera visible above iris (sunset eyes); retinal papilledema.
- Prominent scalp veins and shiny, taut skin; head lag after 4–6 months.
- May exhibit attention deficit, hyperactivity, mental retardation.

- **Clinical indicators of ↑ intracranial pressure.**
  - Infant: Projectile vomiting unassociated with feeding; altered feeding behaviors; irritability; high shrill cry; seizures.
  - Older child: Headache usually in AM, confusion, apathy, ↓ LOC.

Treatment
- Surgical removal of obstruction.
- ↓ excessive CSF by shunting fluid out of the ventricles and to the peritoneum (ventricular peritoneal shunt); shunt revision as the child grows.

Nursing Care
Preoperative
- Maintain Fowler position to permit gravity drainage of CSF.

Pre- and Postoperative
- Assess VS; take serial measures of head circumference (mark site with pen).
- Assess fontanels for bulging daily.
- Assess for clinical indicators of ↑ ICP
- Support head and neck when holding or moving infant; protect from skin breakdown.
- Keep eyes moist and free from irritation.
- Provide small frequent feedings and schedule care around feedings to ↓ vomiting.

Postoperative
- Place on unoperative side to ↓ pressure on shunt; keep flat to prevent rapid decrease in intracranial fluid that may → subdural hematoma.
- Assess for S&S of infection such as shunt malfunction, fever, wound or shunt tract inflammation, poor feeding, vomiting, abdominal pain; most common complication 1–2 months after surgery.

Anencephaly

- Most severe form of neural tube defect; absence of both cerebral hemispheres with an intact brainstem; fatal condition.

Signs and Symptoms
- Neonate has small, malformed head and face with thick neck.
- Frequently stillborn or may live only several hours to a few days.
- Death is usually due to respiratory failure.

Nursing Care
- Provide infant with palliative care.
- Support parents as they consider decision to abort if condition is identified in utero; in coping with realization that their infant has a fatal condition; and when considering organ donation.

Cerebral Palsy (CP)

- Impaired movement, posture, muscle tone, coordination.
- May have intellectual, perceptual, language, emotional deficits.
- Multifactorial causes: Cerebral anoxia most significant (traumatic birth), teratogens, brain malformations, intrauterine infections, prematurity, childhood meningitis, toxin exposure.
- Usually diagnosed at end of first year; nonprogressive; most children have average intelligence.

Signs and Symptoms

- Poor head control and failure to smile by 3 months; unable to sit by 8 months.
- Stiff arms and legs; crossed legs **(scissoring)**; floppiness; pushes away or arches back.
- Irritability and crying, persistent primitive reflexes (asymmetric tonic neck, Moro), tongue thrusting and choking after 6 months, walking on toes, ADHD; seizures.
- **Spastic:** Hypertonicity; ↓ balance, posture, coordination; ↓ fine and gross motor skills.
- **Ataxic:** Wide-based gait; poor performance of rapid repetitive movements or use of upper extremities.
- **Dyskinetic-athetoid:** Abnormal involuntary movements **(dyskinesia)**; slow, writhing movements **(athetosis)**.
- Drooling and imperfect articulation **(dysarthria)**.
- Mixed type/dystonic: Spasticity and athetosis.

Treatment

- PT (braces, splints), OT (adaptive equipment), speech therapy.
- Surgery: Tendon lengthening, selective dorsal rhizotomy.
- Medications: Skeletal muscle relaxants, antiseizure, botulinum toxin type A.
- Education: Early intervention; individualized education program (IEP).
- ↑ calories for energy expenditure; ↑ protein for muscle activity; ↑ vitamin B_6 for amino acid metabolism.

Nursing Care

- Teach careful eating to ↓ risk of aspiration; safe environment; helmet use.
- Do not overstimulate; engage in play appropriate for developmental level and ability; be patient with attempts at speech.
- Assist with bowel and bladder training.
- ROM to stretch heel cords and prevent contractures.
- Teach health maintenance and encourage rehab (PT, OT, speech therapy).
- Teach use and care of orthotics, walking aids, adaptive devices.
- Teach side effects of medications.
- Assist parents and child coping with lifelong disability.

Cognitive Impairment (Mental Retardation)

- No characteristic pathology.
- **Multifactorial causes:**
  - *Genetic:* Down and fragile X syndromes, PKU.
  - *Prenatal:* Alcohol and drug use, infection, ↑ folic acid, prematurity, anoxia.
  - *Medical:* Cranial malformations, meningitis, measles, lead poisoning.
- **Degrees of functioning:**
  - *Mild:* IQ 50-70; educable; mental age 8-12 yr; simple reading, writing, math skills; may function in society and have a job.
  - *Moderate:* IQ 35-55; trainable; mental age 3-7 yr; performs ADLs; has social skills; can work in sheltered workshop.
  - *Severe:* IQ 20-40; barely trainable; mental age ≤ 2 yr; requires support-ive long-term care.
  - *Profound:* IQ <25; may attain mental age of ≤ 1 year; requires total care.

Signs and Symptoms

- ↓ functioning in ≥ two areas such as communication, self-care, home liv-ing, social or interpersonal skills, self-direction, functional academic skills.
- ↓ eye contact, ↑ spontaneous activity, nonresponsive to contact.
- Delayed developmental milestones; poor results on standardized tests (Bayley Scales of Infant Development, 2nd ed.; Wechsler Intelligence Scale for Children-III).
- Passive and dependent to aggressive and impulsive.
- Additional problems such as ↑ coordination; impaired motor, hearing, and vision.
- May have seizures, ADHD, mood disorder.

Treatment

- Early identification; early intervention programs.
- Individualized education program; PT, OT, VT.
- Placement in day care, respite program, or long-term care facility.

Nursing Care

Child

- Use simple, concrete communication and a variety of senses.
- Teach tasks step-by-step while slowly removing assistance **(fading).**
- Give positive reinforcement for desired behavior **(shaping).**
- Role-play social behaviors; support independence with ADL; base play on developmental not chronological age.
- Encourage peer groups such as scouting and Special Olympics.
- Explore sexuality issues with parents and patient, such as code of conduct, contraception, sterilization, protection from sexual abuse.

Parents

■ Support parents coping with diagnosis; decision concerning temporary or permanent placement.

Chromosome Disorders

Turner Syndrome

■ Abnormal or missing X chromosome; occurs in females.
■ **S&S:**
   ■ *Infants:* Lymphedema of hands and feet; low posterior hairline.
   ■ *Children:* Webbed neck, short stature, shield-shaped chest.
   ■ *Adolescents/adults:* Undeveloped secondary sex characteristics, amenorrhea, infertile, immature, difficulty with social cues, socially isolated behavior, usually normal intelligence.

Klinefelter Syndrome

■ Extra X chromosome; occurs in males.
■ **S&S:**
   ■ *Infants/children:* No distinct clinical indicators.
   ■ *Adolescents/adults:* Tall, thin, with long legs and arms; deficient secondary sex characteristics; infertile; gynecomastia; variable mental impairment; learning disabilities; behavioral problems such as ↓ impulse control and hyperactivity.

Trisomy 21 (Down Syndrome)

■ Extra chromosome 21; occurs in males and females.
■ **S&S:**
   ■ *Infants/children:* Small head with flat occiput; small nose with flat bridge **(saddle nose)**; inner epicanthic folds; small, low-set ears; short, thick neck; protruding tongue; broad, short hands and feet; transverse palmar crease; hypotonic musculature; hyperflexible; variable mental impairment; congenital anomalies, especially heart; ↓ immune response; difficulty managing oral secretions; ↑ sociability.
   ■ *Adolescents/adults:* Delayed and/or incomplete sexual development; males usually infertile; females may be fertile; sensory problems such as cataracts and ↓ hearing; short stature; overweight.

Nursing Care

Child
- Maintain airway; protect from infection.
- Interact based on developmental level, not chronological age.
- Prepare for lack of pubertal changes; teach about prescribed hormone replacement.

Parents
- Provide emotional support; encourage genetic counseling.
- Help set realistic goals for child; support decision regarding placement.

Skeletal Malformations

Clubfoot (Talipes Equinovarus) and Developmental Dysplasia of Hip (DDH)

Clubfoot (Talipes Equinovarus)
- Foot in plantar flexion (downward) and deviated medially (inward); rigid or flexible.
- Familial tendency, intrauterine crowding, arrested development.

Signs and Symptoms
- Affected foot/feet smaller, shorter heel pad empty with transverse plantar crease.
- Unilateral affected extremity may be shorter with calf atrophy; ↑ risk of hip dysplasia

Treatment
- Serial casts or surgical correction.

Developmental Dysplasia of Hip (DDH)
- Abnormal development of one or more hip with shallow acetabulum, subluxation, and/or dislocation.
- Physiological, mechanical, genetic causes.

Signs and Symptoms
- **Ortolani sign:** ↑ Abduction of affected leg; audible click when abducting and externally rotating affected hip.
- **Galeazzi sign:** Asymmetry of gluteal, popliteal, and thigh folds; apparent shortening of femur.
- **Trendelenburg sign:** Pelvis tilts downward on unaffected side when standing on affected extremity.
- Waddling gait and lordosis when walking.

Treatment
- Brace, serial casts, surgical correction.

Nursing Care for Infant With Clubfoot or DDH
- Ensure casts are reapplied as child grows.
  - Clubfoot: Daily for 2 weeks, then every 1–2 weeks for total of 8–12 weeks.
  - DDH: Hip spica cast changed when needed every 3–6 months.
- Ensure that splint such as Pavlik harness is applied correctly; splint permits some mobility but prevents hip extension and adduction; straps should be checked every 1–2 weeks; worn continuously for 3–5 months.
- Perform neurovascular check: Blanching, warm toes, able to move toes, pedal pulse.
- **Cast care:** Place diaper below edge of cast; apply transparent film dressing to form bridge between cast and skin; apply clothing over cast to prevent stuffing of food or objects down cast; assess for odor that indicates infection.
- **Splint care:** Sponge-bathe; keep straps dry; place diaper below straps; dress in knee socks and undershirt to prevent skin irritation from straps; inspect skin under straps 3 times daily and massage area under straps; feed with head elevated; use football hold when breastfeeding; hold and cuddle infant; provide appropriate toys; involve child in age-appropriate activities.

Scoliosis

- Complex spinal deformity in three planes: Lateral curvature, spinal rotation causes rib asymmetry, and thoracic hypokyphosis.
- Multifactorial causes: No apparent cause (**idiopathic scoliosis**); genetic autosomal dominant trait; spinal trauma; concurrent neuromuscular conditions such as rheumatoid arthritis, dwarfism.
- X-ray confirms deformity.

Signs and Symptoms
- Most seen during preadolescent growth spurt by primary health-care provider or school-based screening.
- Scapular and hip heights are asymmetrical when child is viewed from behind; asymmetry and prominence of rib cage when bending forward.
- One breast may be larger; clothes do not fit well, such as uneven pants legs or crooked skirt hem.

Treatment
- Depends on extent, location, and type of curve.
- Orthotics such as Boston brace or thoracolumbosacral orthosis.

- Spinal fusion for curves greater than 40°.
- Exercises to prevent atrophy of spinal and abdominal muscles.

Nursing Care

- Teach purpose, function, application, and care of appliance.
- Check skin for irritation; skin care; pad skin under brace.
- Assist with clothing to disguise brace; encourage wearing brace for 16–23 hr daily for several years.
- Support expression of feelings; role-play how to deal with reaction of others to brace.

Postoperative

- Assess VS, wound, neurovascular status of extremities.
- Maintain PCA pump or give analgesics routinely, as pain is intense first 48–72 hr.
- Maintain NGT and urinary catheter and assess bowel sounds and urinary output when removed due to risk for paralytic ileus and urinary retention.
- If anterior approach used, institute care related to thoracotomy.
- Encourage isometric exercises progressing to ambulation and ROM.

Juvenile Idiopathic Arthritis

- Infectious agent activates autoimmune inflammation; familial with female predominance between 1–3 and 8–10 yr of age.
- Results in chronic inflammation of synovium with joint effusion ultimately leading to erosion, destruction, fibrosis of articular cartilage, development of adhesions between joint surfaces, ankylosis of joints.
- Demonstrates remissions and exacerbations.

Signs and Symptoms

- Variable; one or more joints involved, joint swelling due to edema, joint effusion, synovial thickening, weakness and fatigue.
- Stiffness in AM and after inactivity and loss of motion due to muscle spasms and joint inflammation; spindle fingers with thick proximal joint and slender tip.
- Joints may be pain-free, tender, or painful.
- Laboratory results such as ↑ erythrocyte sedimentation rate; ↑ C-reactive protein; leukocytosis; presence of antinuclear antibodies; positive rheumatoid factor.
- Systemic arthritis: ↑ temp; rash; intraocular inflammation (uveitis); pericarditis; enlarged liver, spleen, lymph nodes.

Treatment

- Suppress inflammation and pain with nonsteroidal anti-inflammatory drugs (NSAIDs; avoid aspirin to prevent Reye syndrome); slower-acting antirheumatic drugs (SAARDs; such as methotrexate, sulfasalazine, hydroxychloroquine, gold); a biological agent that blocks cytokine tumor necrosis factor interrupting inflammation (etanercept); cytotoxic agents such as cyclophosphamide and azathioprine.
- Corticosteroids used only when other medications are ineffective because of side effects.
- PT and OT to ↑ muscle strength; mobilize joints; prevent and correct deformities; splinting of knees, wrists, hands to ↓ pain and flexion deformities.

Nursing Care

Child

- Teach to take medications as prescribed even during remissions.
- Maintain functional alignment: Positioning, splints, firm mattress, periodic prone position, small pillow under head.
- Apply ordered heat: 10-min warm tub bath in AM; warm packs to joints for 20 min.
- Encourage independence in ADLs; exercise program; incorporate play in the program such as throwing ball, swimming, or riding bike.
- Balance activity/rest.
- *During exacerbations:* Give medications to ↓ pain, rest joints; maintain functional alignment; encourage isometric not isotonic exercises; maintain contact with school and peers; support developing initiative and industry.

Parents

- Support coping with exacerbations, constant discomfort, risk of overindulgence, and seeking alternative therapies.

Infections and Infestations

Disorder and Etiology	Signs and Symptoms	Treatment	Specific Nursing Care
SCABIES			
• Scabies mite burrows into and multiplies in epidermis. • Transmitted by direct contact with infected person, rarely by fomites.	• Inflammatory response. • Papules, vesicles, pustules usually involving hands, wrists, axillae, genitalia, and inner thighs, feet, ankles. • Mite appears as black dot at end of linear, gray-ish brown threadlike burrow.	• Topical scabicide or ivermectin (Stromectol). • Antibiotics for secondary infection.	• Wear gloves and gown. • Contacts treated because time between infestation and S&S is 1–2 months. • Massage cream thoroughly into skin from head to under feet; keep on 8–14 hr; then shampoo and bathe. • Teach pruritus may take 2–3 weeks to subside; contaminated linen and clothing must be washed and dried at high heat.
PEDICULOSIS (Lice)			
• Louse infests head, body, or pubic hair. • Spread by personal articles such as combs, hats, bedding.	• White eggs (nits) attach to base of hair shafts behind ears and at nape of neck. • Intense pruritus due to crawling insect and insect saliva.	• Pediculicide permethrin 1% cream rinse (Nix). • Nit removed with fine-tooth comb.	• Wear gloves to apply pediculicide. • Protect eyes during application. • Remove visible nits with nit comb.

Disorder and Etiology	Signs and Symptoms	Treatment	Specific Nursing Care
PEDICULOSIS (Lice)			
	• Papules due to secondary infections.		• Teach contaminated linen and clothing must be washed and dried at high heat; vacuum rugs, floors, furniture; soak brushes, combs, hats, scarves in pediculicide for 1 hr.
IMPETIGO			
• Skin infection due to *Staphylococcus* or *Streptococcus* organisms; from autoinoculation or infected person. • Superimposed on eczema.	• Reddish macule becomes vesicular and ruptures, leaving superficial, moist erosion. • Lesions dry as honey-colored crusts; pruritus.	• Removal of undermined skin, crusts, and debris. • Topical application of bactericidal ointment. • Systemic antibiotic.	• Teach parents hand hygiene, contact isolation, preventing scratching, gently rubbing lesions to remove crusts before topical antibiotic.
DIAPER DERMATITIS			
• Excoriation of body surfaces that rub together. • Due to excessive heat, moisture, chafing, exposure to urea or stool, soaps, chemicals in wipes.	• Red, inflamed, moist, partially denuded skin at intergluteal folds, groin, neck, axilla. • *Candidiasis:* Scaly, erythematous skin, rash, possibly covered with exudates, painful.	• Keep area clean and dry; expose to air and light; use barrier ointment. • *Candidiasis:* Oral or topical antifungals.	• Bathe area daily, pat dry, keep skin folds separated, expose to air and light several times daily for 20 min. • Use disposable superabsorbent diapers; change often; apply barrier ointment.

Continued

Disorder and Etiology	Signs and Symptoms	Treatment	Specific Nursing Care
DIAPER DERMATITIS			
• Candidiasis (moniliasis) infection with *C. albicans*.			• *Candidiasis:* Teach hand hygiene; give prescribed medications.
RINGWORM			
• Fungal infection of skin. • *Tinea capitis* • Scalp, hairline, neck. • *Tinea cruris (jock itch)* Inner thigh, crural fold, scrotum in men. • *T. capitis* and *T. cruris* Transmitted person-to-person, animal-to-person, via contaminated items. • *Tinea pedis (athlete's foot)* Between toes or plantar surface of feet; often transmitted in locker room.	• Pruritus, characteristic lesions. • *Tinea capitis* • Patchy, scaly areas of alopecia. • *Tinea cruris* • Round, erythematous, scaling patch. • *Tinea pedis* • Maceration, fissures, small vesicles.	• Oral griseofulvin. • Local application of antifungal. • *Tinea capitis* • Selenium shampoos.	• Teach personal hygiene. • Avoid pets, particularly cats. • Avoid sharing personal items such as combs and hats. • Wear plastic shoes in swimming areas and locker rooms. • Wear cotton socks and underwear, ventilated shoes, to ↓ heat and perspiration.

Viral Infections

Disorder and Etiology	Signs and Symptoms	Treatment	Specific Nursing Care
VERRUCA (WARTS)			
• Caused by human papillomavirus. • *V. plantaris*—plantar wart. • *V. vulgaris*—limited to epidermis.	• ***Warts*** • Gray or brown, elevated papules mostly on hands, face, soles of feet (plantar wart). • Unpredictable course; may disappear spontaneously.	• ***Warts and Molluscum Contagiosum*** • Removed by curettage, electrocautery, cryotherapy, caustic solutions.	• Teach to avoid skin-to-skin contact. • Encourage frequent hand hygiene. • Give prescribed medications.
MOLLUSCUM CONTAGIOSUM			
• Pox virus. • Spread by skin-to-skin, fomite-to-skin, autoinoculation.	• ***Molluscum Contagiosum*** • May be asymptomatic; flesh-colored papules. • May spontaneously resolve.		
HERPES VIRUS TYPE I, SIMPLEX OR TYPE II, GENITAL			
• Transmitted via respiratory droplets, virus containing fluids such as saliva or cervical secretions (vaginal birth and sexual contact).	• ***Herpes Virus Type I and II*** • Itching, burning vesicles near lips, nose, genitals, buttocks; forms crust, then exfoliates. • Spontaneous healing in 8–10 days; may be fatal in child with ↓ immunity.	• ***Herpes Virus—Type I and II*** • Topical or systemic antivirals; topical anesthetic; sunscreen to ↓ risk. • ***Herpes Virus—Type II*** • Cesarean birth if mother has active lesions.	

Integumentary System Problems

Atopic Dermatitis (Eczema)

- Symmetric cutaneous inflammation with erythema, papules, vesicles, pustules, scales, crusts, scabs; may be dry or have a weeping discharge; secondary infections common.
- Multifactorial causes: Genetics, stress, abnormal function of skin such as alterations in perspiration, peripheral vascular function, heat tolerance; environmental factors such as dry climate, exacerbations in fall and winter; IgE food sensitization; T-cell dysfunction resulting in allergy to dust, mold, animal hair, and chemicals.

Signs and Symptoms

- Characteristic lesions on cheeks, scalp, neck, flexor surface of arms and legs.
- Intense itching or burning, facial pallor, bluish discoloration beneath eyes **(allergic shiners)**.
- S&S of secondary infections. Diagnosis based on history and morphological findings.

Treatment

- Depends on cause; topical lotions to hydrate skin; colloid tub baths; phototherapy with ultraviolet light; avoid precipitating agent.
- Antihistamines; topical steroids; topical or systemic immunosuppressants; interferons; essential fatty acids; topical pimecrolimus (Elide); systemic antibiotics for skin infections.

Nursing Care

Child

- Hydrate skin: Short bath with mild soap such as Neutrogena or Dove and immediately lubricate moist skin (Eucerin, Aquaphor, Cetaphil).
- ↑ itching and scratching: Short nails filed to remove edges; cotton socks on hands and pinned to shirt; soft cotton fabrics; moderate environmental temperatures; teach S&S of secondary infection.
- Avoid irritants: Harsh soap, fabric softeners, bubble baths, excessive bathing, rough and woolen fabrics; double-rinse clothing after washing.
- Allergy-proof home: No rugs, drapes, down pillows, wool blankets; wet dust and vacuum when child is out of house.
- Hypoallergenic diet: Teach diet; introduce one food at a time.

Parent

- Cuddle irritable child coping with itching; teach that condition is not communicable and scars generally will not occur if secondary infections are prevented.

Burns

For additional information, see Tab 6, MEDSURG, Burns, p. 187.

Estimating Extent of Injury
- Total body surface area (TBSA) injured represented as a percentage of body surface.
- Modified rule of nines by %:
  - Head and neck are 18%.
  - Anterior trunk is 18%.
  - Posterior trunk is 18%.
  - Each arm is 9%.
  - Each leg is 14%.
  - For each year of life after 2, 1% is deducted from head and 0.5% is added to each leg until adult percentages are reached.

Fluid Replacement Therapy
- Initiated for burns >15%–20% TBSA.
- Parkland formula often used.
- IVF to maintain urine output of 1–2 mL/kg for child weighing <30 kg and 30–50 mL/hr in older child.
- Urinary output, capillary refill, and sensorium are used to evaluate hydration status and fluid replacement needs.

Nursing Care
Child
- Medicate before painful procedures; explain treatments are not punishments.
- Provide age-appropriate support; allow choices whenever possible.
- Encourage expression of feelings; young children coping with separation anxiety and adolescents developing an identity are most affected.
- Assist coping with physical changes; compression bandages and splints; reactions of peers.
- Accept regression; use behavior modification to motivate.
- Teach age-appropriate fire safety information such as stop, drop, and roll if clothing is on fire; not playing with matches, outlets, or stoves.

Parents
- Support coping with critically ill child; guilt; helplessness; concerns for child's physical and emotional future.
- Explain multidisciplinary follow-up as scar tissue will require grafts; reconstructive surgery; PT & OT.

Poisoning

Chemical	Signs & Symptoms	Treatment	Nursing Care
HYDROCARBONS			
Kerosene, gasoline, turpentine, furniture polish, cleaning fluids.	• Coughing, gagging, N&V, lethargy, ↓ R, cyanosis, substernal retractions, grunting.	• Gastric lavage with endotracheal tube to prevent aspiration. • IVF oxygen.	• Never induce vomiting to avoid further damage. • Assess VS and oral mucous membranes for clinical indicators of burns. • Maintain patent airway. • Give ordered oxygen and medications.
CORROSIVE CHEMICALS			
Bleach, oven, or drain cleaners; detergents; electric dishwasher granules.	• Severe burning in oral cavity and stomach. • White, swollen mucous membranes; edema of lips, tongue, pharynx; vomiting, hemoptysis, hematemesis. • Anxiety, agitation.	• NPO, IVF, analgesics, oxygen, and endotracheal tube prn. • Repeated dilations or surgery for esophageal stricture.	

Chemical	Signs & Symptoms	Treatment	Nursing Care
LEAD (Plumbism)			
• Lead in paint, soil, dust, drinking water.	• Blood concentration >10 mg/100 mL, anemia, pallor, fatigue. • Lead line on teeth and long bones. • Joint pain, headache, lethargy, irritability, hyperactivity, insomnia, seizures.	• Chelation therapy when blood lead level nears 45 mcg/dL.	• Screen at 1–2 yr; routinely if high risk. • Eliminate source. • Ensure adequacy of urinary output before chelation therapy.
ACETAMINOPHEN			
• Most common medication poisoning in children. • History of 150 mg/kg for several days.	• N&V, diaphoresis, ↓ urine output, pallor, weakness, bradycardia, liver failure, RUQ pain, coagulation abnormalities, jaundice, confusion, and coma.	• Assess for S&S of liver failure. • Activated charcoal if ingestion ≤1 hr; if >1 hr, N-acetylcysteine in loading dose, then 17 maintenance doses. • Oral or IV fluids.	• Give prescribed antidote. • Teach medication regimen. • Give ordered oral and IV fluids.
SALICYLATE (ASA)			
Toxicity Acute • 300–500 mg/kg/day **Chronic** • >100 mg/kg/day	• Diaphoresis, N&V, oliguria, ↑T, hyperpnea, tinnitus, dizziness, delirium. • **Poisoning:** Confusion, metabolic acidosis, hyperventilation, and coma.	• Gastric lavage, activated charcoal, saline cathartics. • IVF, vitamin K if bleeding. • Peritoneal dialysis, hypothermia blanket prn.	• Assess VS. • Maintain airway and ventilation. • Give prescribed medications, IVF. • Provide care when on hypothermia blanket or receiving dialysis.

Nursing Care for Children With Poisoning
Emergency Care
■ Identify agent; stop exposure; do not induce vomiting—may redamage mucosa; prevent aspiration; flush eyes and skin with water if involved.
■ Call American Association of Poison Control Centers for directions.
■ Transport to hospital; bring evidence such as container and vomitus.

Acute Care
■ Ensure airway; assess VS, hepatic and renal function; do not scold child or parent.

Prevention
■ Teach child not to eat nonfood items **(pica)**; obey parent's safety rules.
■ Teach parents to keep toxins and drugs in locked cabinet; use childproof containers.

Light Therapy (Phototherapy)
Electroconvulsive Therapy (ECT)
Seclusion and Restraint
Occupational Therapy
Activity Therapy
Crisis Intervention
Psychopharmacology

Legal and Ethical Issues Overview

- **Voluntary admission/commitment:** Patient consents to admission; free to leave even against medical advice.
- **Emergency commitment:** Without patient consent when a danger to self or others or is gravely disabled; assessed by two mental health professionals; probable cause hearing must take place within 5 days where convincing evidence must be produced to continue in- or outpatient treatment.
- **Civil or judicial commitment:** Longer than emergency commitment to provide treatment (parens patriae: state power to protect or care for patients with disabilities or to protect public); rules vary by state; generally renewable in 90 days or 6 months.
- **Right to least restrictive environment:** Restraints or seclusion cannot be used until less-restrictive interventions are tried first.
- **Confidentiality:** Health Insurance Portability and Accountability Act (HIPAA) of 1996 guarantees privacy and security of health information and enforcement standards; psychotherapy and substance abuse treatment have additional privacy protection.
- **Competency:** Patient capable of making decisions about treatment.
- **Informed consent:** Right to know risks and benefits to make decisions.
- **Reporting laws:** Nurses must report suspected child and elder abuse or neglect; warn a person and those able to protect a person about a threat made to kill them even if it breaches confidentiality.

Nursing Care

- Know federal and state regulations and standards regarding legal issues and relationship to information management.
- Employ advocacy role.
- Inform and protect patient's rights, such as provide information for informed consent, accept right to refuse treatment or medications.
- Maintain confidentiality; consult with agency attorney before releasing information about patient to others or secure signed release from patient.

- Enact duty to warn patient's potential intended victims.
- Support least restrictive environment, including decreased use of chemical restraints; refer to Joint Commission and federal and state standards.
- Know signs and symptoms (S&S) of child and elder abuse such as bruises, burns, injuries, inconsistent reporting, signs of sexual abuse, old fractures; exaggerated, absent, hostile or emotional response of caregiver; signs of failure to thrive.

Mental Health Assessment

- **Stressors:** Assess internal and external stressors.
- **Appearance:** Note grooming, hygiene, posture, eye contact, clothing. Is appearance congruent with developmental stage and age?
- **General attitude:** Is patient cooperative or uncooperative; ingratiating, friendly, or distant; hostile, open or defensive, passive, resistive?
- **Activity and behavior:** Congruent with feelings? Note mannerisms, gestures, gait. Is patient restless, agitated, or calm? Is activity hyperactive, aggressive, rigid, or relaxed? Are there tremors, tics?
- **Sensory and cognitive status:** Assess level of consciousness; orientation to person, place, time; recall, recent, and remote memory; confusion; ability to concentrate.
- **Thought processes:** Is thinking rapid, slow, or repetitious? How long is the patient's attention span? Assess content: Is patient delusional, suicidal, obsessive, paranoid, phobic, or expressing religiosity or magical thinking? How is the patient's thinking disorganized? Assess for echolalia, tangentiality, confabulation, loose associations, concrete thinking, clang associations, referential thinking, circumstantiality, and neologisms.
- **Judgment and insight:** Assess decision-making, problem-solving, and coping ability. Can patient manage activities of daily living? Does patient understand the concepts of cause and effect?
- **Mood:** Is patient emotionally labile, depressed, sad, happy, anxious, fearful, irritable, euphoric, guilty, despairing, apathetic, angry, shameful, proud, relieved, content, confident, or bizarre?
- **Affect (ability to vary emotional expression):** Is patient's affect congruent with mood or is it flat or inappropriate?
- **Speech:** Are volume and rate congruent with feelings and behavior? Is there pressured speech or aphasia?
- **Self-concept and self-esteem:** Does patient make negative or positive statements about self? What is the extent of patient's satisfaction with self and/or body image?
- **Perception:** Is patient experiencing hallucinations, illusions, or depersonalization?

- **Impulse control:** Does patient exhibit disinhibition, aggression, hyperactivity, hypersexuality, or inappropriate social behavior?
- **Potential for violence:** Are there signs of risk for violence such as depression, suicidal ideation, increased muscle tension, pacing, profanity, and verbal and/or physical threats?
- **Family and social systems:** What is patient's attainment and maintenance of interpersonal relationships and extent of support system?
- **Spiritual status:** Note patient's presence or absence of and comfort with beliefs, values, and religious affiliation.

Defense Mechanisms

Defense Mechanism	Example
Compensation: Increase capabilities in one area to make up for deficiencies in another.	Nonathletic student joins debate team.
Denial: Ego unable to accept painful reality.	Person assumes false cheerfulness or fails to seek medical help when needed.
Displacement: Directing anger toward less-threatening substitute.	Patient yells at a significant other after being diagnosed with cancer.
Intellectualization: Situation dealt with on cognitive, not emotional, level.	Patient discusses all test results but avoids focusing on fears and feelings.
Projection: Attaching to others feelings that are unacceptable to self.	Preoperative patient says to wife, "Don't be scared."
Rationalization: Attempt to logically justify or excuse unacceptable behaviors.	Mother of a latchkey 10-yr-old says, "He needs to learn to be self-sufficient."
Reaction formation: Opposite reaction to the way one really feels.	A person does not like a neighbor but is overly friendly.
Regression: Retreat to an earlier, more comfortable developmental age.	Adolescent has a temper tantrum when told not to do something.

Defense Mechanism	Example
Repression: Unconscious blocking of unacceptable thoughts from the conscious mind.	A woman has no recollection of her father's sexual abuse.
Suppression: Conscious blocking of thoughts from the mind.	Patient states, "I'll worry about that after my test tomorrow."
Undoing: Action or words cancel previous action or words to decrease guilt.	Husband gives wife a gift after abusing her.

Review of Mental Health Disorders

Alzheimer's Disease

Stage 1: Mild
- Patient recognizes a problem.
- ↓ short-term memory, mild cognition impairment, confusion, hyperalertness.
- Anxiety; depression; invents words that have no common meaning (**neologisms**).
- Fills in memory gaps with invented facts (**confabulation**).

Stage 2: Moderate
- Intellectual decline continues; language disturbance (**aphasia**).
- ↓ motor activity (**apraxia**).
- Failure to recognize words/objects (**agnosia**).
- Repetition of same idea in response to different stimuli (**perseveration**).
- Confusion/irritation at end of day (**sundowning**); sleep disturbances with wandering.
- Acting on thoughts/feelings without social control (**disinhibition**).
- Agitation, aggression, illusions, delusions, and hallucinations.

Stage 3: Severe
- Totally dependent; complete loss of intellectual functioning.
- Difficulty swallowing (**dysphagia**); emaciation; ↓ bowel and bladder control.
- Immobility leads to pneumonia, urinary tract infections, and pressure ulcers.

Anorexia and Bulimia

Signs & Symptoms

	Behavioral	Physical	Psychological
Anorexia	• Self-starvation. • Rituals regarding food, eating. • Weight loss. • Behaviors to ↓ weight: purging, exercise, use of laxatives, enemas, and diuretics.	• Weight loss 15% below ideal. • Cachexia (sunken eyes, protruding bones, dry skin). • Amenorrhea. • Decreased pulse and body temperature. • Lanugo on face. • Constipation. • Sensitivity to cold.	• Appears fat to self. • Intense, irrational fear of being fat. • Preoccupation with cooking, food, nutrition. • Delayed psychosexual development. • Perfectionist, high achiever.
Bulimia	• Repetitive secret bingeing and purging. • Behaviors to ↓ weight: purging, exercise, use of laxatives, enemas, and diuretics. • Fasts to compensate for bingeing.	• Weight usually is normal; may be higher or lower. • Fluid and electrolyte imbalances such as hypokalemia, metabolic alkalosis, dehydration. • Lack of control over eating during bingeing. • Menstrual irregularities. • Dental caries, loss of dental enamel. • Hypotension, cardiac dysrhythmias. • Constipation or diarrhea. • GERD, parotid enlargement.	• Excessive concern about weight, shape, proportions. • Depression, shame, self-contempt follow bingeing. • Mood swings, irritability. • Impulsive, extrovert.

Anxiety Disorders

Generalized Anxiety
■ Excessive anxiety for 6 months; hypervigilance; difficult to control worry.
■ Three or more of the following S&S:
  ■ Restlessness, irritability
  ■ Tachycardia, chest tightness
  ■ Easily fatigued
  ■ Sleep disturbance
  ■ Tremors
  ■ Increased muscle tension
  ■ Diaphoresis
  ■ Dizziness
  ■ Decreased concentration

Panic
■ Panic attacks lasting from 10–30 min (see Levels of Anxiety and Related S&S, next page).
■ Unrealistic fear of objects, activities, and situations such as heights (**acrophobia**), open spaces (**agoraphobia**).

Post-Traumatic Stress Disorder (PTSD)
■ Precipitated by a traumatic event; hypervigilance; persistent anxiety.
■ **Acute:** S&S first evident <3 months after the event.
■ **Chronic:** S&S first evident >3 months after the event.
■ **Delayed:** S&S first evident >6 months after the event.
■ Flashbacks; nightmares; anniversary reactions.

Levels of Anxiety and Related S&S

Factor	Mild	Moderate	Severe	Panic
Perception	Broad, alert.	Narrowed, focused.	Greatly narrowed, selective attention.	Distorted, scattered.
Motor activity	Slight muscle tension.	↑ muscle tension, tremors.	Extreme muscle tension, ↑ motor activity.	Erratic behavior, combative or withdrawn.
Communication	Questioning.	Pitch changes, voice tremors.	Difficulty communicating.	Incoherent.
Mood	Relaxed, calm.	Energized, nervous.	Irritable, extremely upset.	Panicky, angry, terrified.
Physiological responses	Normal vital signs (VS).	Slight ↑ in pulse and respirations.	Fight or flight response: ↑VS, dilated pupils, hyperventilation, headache, diaphoresis, nausea, diarrhea, urgency, frequency.	Continuation of fight or flight response; may exhibit dyspnea, pallor, hypotension.
Learning	Enhanced, uses learning to adapt.	Impaired, focuses on one issue, selective attention.	Greatly diminished, improbable, ↓ concentration, ↑ distractibility.	Impossible, unable to learn.

Attention Deficit and Disruptive Behavior Disorders

Disorder	Description
Attention deficit hyperactivity disorder (ADHD)	Usually identified before age 7; occurs in at least two settings such as social, academic, work. **Persistent inattention**: Careless; easily distracted; forgetful; loses things; does not finish tasks; ↓ concentration; ↓ organization. **Hyperactivity**: Runs, climbs, talks, fidgets excessively; impulsive; ↓ ability to wait for turn.
Oppositional defiant disorder	Pattern of disobedience and/or hostile behavior toward authority figures.
Conduct disorder	Pattern of aggressive, destructive behavior with disregard for others and norms of society.

Cognitive Disorders

Disorder	Description
Delirium	Acute ↓ cognition, lability, fear, delusions, ↑ P, ↑ R, ↑ BP, hallucinations, illusions, disorientation, dilated pupils, diaphoresis, sleep disturbances, tremor; may be reversible if due to metabolic imbalance or drug withdrawal.
Dementia	Intellectual decline such as ↓ short-term memory, language, insight, and judgment; self-preoccupation; may be passive such as flat affect and ↓ spontaneity OR irritable such as sarcastic, ↓ concern for others, paranoid; progresses from mild to severe; patient ultimately needs total care.

Dissociative Disorders

Disorder	Description
Dissociative identity	Coexistence of two or more distinct personalities within one person.
Depersonalization	Persistent and recurrent feelings of detachment from one's body and thoughts.
Dissociative fugue	Sudden unexpected travel with ↓ ability to recall one's identity or past; or assumption of new identity.
Dissociative amnesia	Memory loss related to an acute, precipitating traumatic event.
Malingering	Fabricating a false or exaggerated symptom to gain attention; assumes sick role.
Munchausen syndrome	Intentionally causes own illness, sabotages diagnostic tests. **By proxy:** Parent creates illness in child and then seeks treatment to gain attention.

Mood Disorders

Disorder	Signs and Symptoms
Bipolar: manic and hypomanic episodes	Elevated, irritable mood for 4 days (**hypomanic**) or 1 week (**manic**) alternating with depression plus 3 or more of the following: ↓ sleep, grandiosity, flight of ideas, pressured speech, ↑ goal-directed activity, distractibility, ↑ pleasurable activities with negative results such as buying sprees.
Depressive episodes	Depressed mood for 2 weeks plus 5 or more of the following: ↓↑ weight, ↑↓ sleep, psychomotor agitation or retardation, feelings of worthlessness, inappropriate guilt, ↓ concentration, suicidal ideation.
Major depression	Depressed mood for ≥2 weeks, ↓ pleasure (**anhedonia**) plus 4 or more of the following: ↑↓ appetite, ↓↑ weight, psychomotor agitation or retardation, altered sleep, ↓ concentration, ↓ energy, suicidal ideation.

Disorder	Signs and Symptoms
Dysthymic	Mild, chronic major depression lasting ≥2 yr.
Cyclothymic	Moderate depression to hypomania that may or may not include periods of normal mood lasting ≥2 yr.
Postpartum blues	Unstable mood such as anxiety, fatigue, and/or weepiness first 14 days after birth of child; resolves spontaneously.
Postpartum depression	Unstable mood such as anxiety, insomnia, ↓ energy, ↓ concentration, and/or despair about perceived maternal inadequacies 3–12 months after birth of child.
Postpartum psychosis	Rapid onset 2–6 weeks after birth of child; includes insomnia, agitation, hallucinations, bizarre feelings and behavior, and/or risk for harm to infant.

Personality Disorders

	Cluster A
Paranoid	Suspicious, fearful, irritable, stubborn, uses projection, hyperalert, aloof, argumentative.
Schizoid	Loner, blunted affect, vague thoughts **(poverty of thought)**, indifferent to others.
Schizotypal	Eccentric behavior, appearance, speech; inappropriate affect; indecisive; withdrawn.
	Cluster B
Borderline personality	Unstable relationships, impulsive, intense mood swings, identity disturbance, self-destructive behavior, views things as all good or all bad **(dichotomous thinking)**.
Antisocial personality	Manipulates and exploits others without guilt; lying, stealing, aggressive; seeks attention and immediate gratification; does not learn from mistakes.
Histrionic personality	Emotional instability, hyperexcitability, attention getting, vain, manipulative, dramatic.
Narcissistic personality	Grandiosity, need for attention and admiration, egocentric, arrogant, vain, perfectionist, disturbed relationships, lability of mood.

Continued

	Cluster C
Avoidant personality	Social discomfort, timidity, loner, fear of embarrassment, hurt by criticism.
Dependent personality	Dependent, submissive, indecisive, decreased self-concept, fears rejection.
Obsessive-compulsive	Recurrent, intrusive thoughts **(obsessive)**; driven, repetitive rituals **(compulsive)**; regards self as all-powerful **(omnipotent)** and all-knowing **(omniscient)**.
Not otherwise specified	Mixed components of personality disorders: **Depressive:** Dejected mood, decreased self-esteem, negative, feelings of guilt and remorse. **Passive-aggressive:** Passively resists responsibilities, envious and resentful of others, sullen, psychomotor agitation/retardation, argumentative, procrastinator.

Pervasive Developmental Disorders

Asperger syndrome	Normal IQ; exceptional talent in one area **(savant)**; interpersonal awkwardness; viewed as eccentric; may have bizarre obsessions.
Autistic (autism)	Avoids eye contact; dislikes being touched; may whirl, rock, toe walk; slow language development; rigid; tantrums; abnormal speech pattern; repetitive behaviors or words **(perseveration)**; may self-mutilate; may be a savant.

Sexual and Gender Identity Disorders

Sexual disorders	Decreased sexual desire: e.g., avoidance of genital contact. Decreased sexual arousal: e.g., ↓ ability to attain and/or maintain sexual excitement/erection. Orgasmic: e.g., delay/absence of orgasm after excitement, premature ejaculation; female sexual painful intercourse **(dyspareunia)**, involuntary perineal muscle contraction with intercourse **(vaginismus)**.

Gender identity	Persistent discomfort with birth gender; desire to change sex characteristics or gender; cross-dressing.
Paraphilias	Sexual arousal by: **Pedophilia:** Sexual activity with child. **Exhibitionism:** Genital exposure to stranger. **Frotteurism:** Touching nonconsenting person. **Fetishism:** Use of an object. **Voyeurism:** Watching unsuspecting nakedness or sexual activity. **Sadism:** Inflicting suffering and/or humiliation on another. **Masochism:** Self-humiliation and/or suffering.

Schizophrenia

- Mental disorder characterized by disturbances in form and content of thought, mood, affect, behavior, and sense of self.
- Two or more of the positive and negative symptoms for 6 months must be present.

Positive Symptoms: Type I
- **Delusion:** Fixed false belief without external stimulus.
- **Hallucination:** False sensory perception without external stimulus.
- Excess or distortion of normal functions (see Disorganized Thinking and Disorganized Behavior, p. 160).

Negative Symptoms: Type II
- Decrease or loss of normal functions.
- **Affective flattening:** ↓ in range and intensity of emotion.
- **Alogia:** ↓ fluency and productivity of thoughts and speech.
- **Ambivalence:** Indecisive because of strong opposing feelings.
- **Anhedonia:** Inability to experience pleasure.
- **Avolition:** Unable to initiate/persist in goal-directed behavior.

Neurocognitive Impairments Associated With Schizophrenia
- Neurocognitive impairments may occur independent of positive and negative symptoms; however, most are positive symptoms.
- Impairments consist of disorganized thinking and disorganized behavior.

Disorganized Thinking

- **Concrete thinking:** Lack of abstraction.
- **Circumstantiality:** Detailed, long discussion about a topic.
- **Clang association:** Repetition of similar-sounding words.
- **Echolalia:** Parrotlike repetition of another's words.
- **Flight of ideas:** Rapid, repeated change in topics.
- **Ideas of reference:** Remarks unrelated to the individual are interpreted personally by the individual.
- **Loose associations:** Decreased connectedness of thoughts and topics.
- **Neologisms:** Made-up words with no common meaning.
- **Pressured speech:** Rapid, forced speech.
- **Tangentiality:** Logical digression from original discussion.

Disorganized Behavior

- **Agitation:** Restlessness with increased emotions/tension.
- **Aggression:** Hostility with potential for verbal or physical violence.
- **Psychomotor disturbances:**
  - **Stereotypy:** Repetitive, purposeless activity peculiar to patient.
  - **Echopraxia:** Involuntary imitation of another's gestures.
  - **Waxy flexibility:** Fixed posturing for extended periods.
- **Regressed behavior:** Childlike, immature behavior.
- **Hypervigilance:** Sustained increased attention to external stimuli.

Schizophrenia (Specific Types)

- **Paranoid:** Delusions of persecution, grandiosity, religiosity, or somatization; disorganized thinking/behavior.
- **Disorganized:** Childlike affect, socially inept, disorganized speech/behavior, sexually uninhibited.
- **Catatonic:** Psychomotor disturbance that may be excessive or involve waxy flexibility, negativism, mutism, posturing, echolalia, echopraxia.
- **Undifferentiated:** Delusions, hallucinations, disorganized speech and behavior.

Somatoform Disorders

Body dysmorphic	Preoccupation with real or imagined defect in appearance; hinders work and social functioning.
Somatization	Physical symptoms without an underlying organic basis.
Conversion	Anxiety unconsciously converted to physical symptoms, rigid, orderly.
Hypochondriasis	Abnormal concern about perceived physical symptoms and health despite absence of illness.

Substance Abuse Disorders

Substance Abuse
- **Dependence:** Craving for substance; failure to meet roles; legal problems; impaired relationships; substance-specific S&S; continued use of substance despite consequences.
- **Intoxication:** Reversible substance-specific syndrome due to recent use.
- **Tolerance:** Increased dose needed for same result.
- **Polysubstance abuse:** Abuse of two or more substances.
- **Potentiation:** Two or more substances produce effect more than sum of each.
- **Withdrawal:** Substance-specific syndrome due to decreased intake or cessation.

Alcohol Abuse
- Excessive, episodic, solitude, and/or morning drinking; slurring; decreased memory; aggressive; blackouts; decreased coordination.
- **Korsakoff psychosis:** Delirium, confabulation, illusions, decreased short/long-term memory, hallucinations.
- **Wernicke encephalopathy:** Neurological abnormalities such as oculomotor dysfunction, confusion, and ataxia due to decreased thiamine.
- **Withdrawal:** Begins in 12 hr, peaks in 48–72 hr, improves by fourth to fifth day; nausea and vomiting (N&V), ↑ VS, diaphoresis, anxiety, restlessness, illusions, hallucinations, tremors, gastrointestinal (GI) disturbances; withdrawal delirium **(delirium tremens)** may occur on 2nd but as late as 14th day.

Opiates (Heroin, Codeine)
- Euphoria; sedation; constricted pupils, constipation; decreased libido, memory, and concentration.
- **Withdrawal:** GI cramps, rhinorrhea, watery eyes, dilated pupils, yawning, nausea, diarrhea, diaphoresis.

Stimulants (Amphetamines, Cocaine)
- Euphoria, initial central nervous system (CNS) stimulation, then depression, insomnia, ↓ appetite, dilated pupils, tremors, paranoia, aggressiveness.
- **Withdrawal:** First psychomotor retardation, then agitation; dysphoria; fatigue and insomnia; cravings; increased appetite; vivid, unpleasant dreams.

Other Abused Substances
- Nicotine; caffeine; hallucinogens (e.g., lysergic acid diethylamide [LSD]); cannabis (e.g., marijuana, hashish); inhalants (e.g., glue, lighter fluid).
- CNS depressants (e.g., sedatives and anxiolytics); phencyclidine (PCP).

Grief and Loss

- **Grief:** Subjective state of emotional, physical, and social responses to the loss of something valued; it may be real, substantiated by others (e.g., death of a loved one); it may be perceived, not identified by others (e.g., loss of masculinity after a prostatectomy).
- **Anticipatory grief:** Work of grieving happens before the loss occurs.
- **Complicated grief:** Secondary to multiple losses such as traumatic death or loss of partner; social isolation; substance abuse; morbid focus on deceased; suicidal thoughts; >3–6 months.
- **Delayed or inhibited grief:** Absence of S&S of grief when loss occurs due to culture, denial, ↓ resources to cope with loss, ↑ need to resume role.

Kübler-Ross Stages of Grieving

Stage and Responses	Nursing Care
Denial: "Not me"; unable to believe loss; may exhibit cheerfulness.	• Explore own feelings about death and dying. Accept but do not strengthen denial. • Encourage communication.
Anger: "Why me?"; questioning; resists loss with hostility/anger.	• Recognize anger is a form of coping. • Do not abandon patient or become defensive. • Help others to understand patient's anger.
Bargaining: "Yes, me, but"; barters for time and may express guilt for past behavior.	• Assist with ventilation of feelings such as guilt, fear, sadness. • Help with unfinished business if appropriate.
Depression: "Yes, me"; realizes full impact; grieves future losses; may talk, withdraw, cry, or feel extremely lonely.	• Convey caring; use touch; sit quietly. • Acknowledge sad feelings. • Accept and support grieving.
Acceptance: "OK, me"; accepts loss; may have decreased interest in activities and people; may be quiet or peaceful.	• Support completion of personal affairs. • Support family participation in care. • Do not abandon patient and family. • Help family understand and allow patient's withdrawal.

Nursing Care for Patients Who Are Grieving

- Assess for stage of grieving; identify expected grieving behaviors; provide adequate time to grieve.
- Encourage verbalization of feelings such as fears, helplessness, anger, guilt.
- Review events of the loss to help patient actualize the loss.
- Identify use of unhealthy defenses such as substance abuse, social isolation, somatic concerns.
- Support honest review of the loss by patient; promote review of positive and negative aspects.
- Support cultural and spiritual rituals associated with the loss.
- Help to identify personal, social, and community support systems.
- Encourage patient to seek grief counseling or attend support group if desired.

Nursing Care of Patients With Mental Health Problems

General Nursing Care for All Patients

- Maintain safe, supportive, nonjudgmental environment.
- Recognize all behavior has meaning.
- Encourage ventilation of feelings; do not deny or approve.
- Accept and respect patients as individuals; provide choices when able.
- Set simple, fair, consistent expectations and limits about behavior; address inappropriate behavior immediately.
- Help patient to test new interpersonal skills.
- Assist with ADLs as necessary.
- Encourage activities that involve patient in recovery.
- Teach patient and family members about prescribed medications.

Nursing Care for Patients With Addictions

- Repeated and chronic use of a substance resulting in dependency.
- Associated with substance abuse, antisocial personality.
- Use screening tools to assess risk; assess for S&S of specific addiction.
- Limit noise and light to decrease hallucinations and illusions due to withdrawal.
- Provide and encourage maintenance of a substance-free setting.
- Accept hostility without reprisal; set realistic limits to decrease manipulation and/or aggression.

- Expect patient to assume responsibility for own behavior.
- Encourage patient and family members to attend self-help groups.
- Help family members to identify and change enabling behaviors.

Assessment of Risk for Alcohol Abuse

	CAGE Questionnaire
C	Have you ever felt that you should Cut down on your drinking?
A	Have people Annoyed you by criticizing your drinking?
G	Have you ever felt Guilty about your drinking?
E	Have you ever had a drink in the morning as an Eye-opener?

Nursing Care for Patients Who Are Aggressive

- Hostile verbal, symbolic, or physical behavior that intimidates others.
- Associated with substance abuse, conduct disorders, mania, delirium, dementia, paranoid schizophrenia.
- Assign to a single room; use nonthreatening body language and calm approach; respect personal space; do not touch.
- Provide ongoing surveillance; position self near an escape route; know where colleagues are if help is needed.
- Remove potentially violent or violent patient from vicinity of others.
- Anticipate needs to decrease stress that may cause anger.
- Assess for frustration, irritation, anger, distorted thinking that may precede violence.
- Assist to express anger in acceptable ways such as words, writing list of grievances, physical exercise, assertiveness; provide positive reinforcement for acceptable behavior.
- Teach to interrupt aggressive patterns such as count to 10 or remove self.

Nursing Care for Patients Who Are Anxious

- Anxiety ranges from feelings of apprehension to doom; response to a perceived threat to physiological, emotional, or social integrity.
- Associated with phobias and anxiety, obsessive-compulsive, dissociative, and somatoform disorders.
- Assess level of anxiety.

- Provide single room; decrease environmental stimuli.
- Acknowledge feelings about phobic object or situation.
- Recognize somatic complaints but do not call attention to them.
- Assist to identify and avoid anxiety-producing situations.
- Assist with relaxation techniques to decrease anxiety.
- Postpone teaching when anxiety reaches severe or panic levels.
- Stay with patient during a panic attack; provide for safety.
- Intervene when acting-out impulses may harm self or others.

Nursing Care for Patients With Delusions or Hallucinations

- **Delusion:** Fixed false belief without external stimulus.
  - Types: grandiosity, persecution, control, religiosity, erotomanic, somatic, ideas of reference, thought broadcasting, withdrawal, and insertion.
- **Hallucination:** False sensory perception without external stimulus.
  - Types: auditory, visual, gustatory, olfactory, tactile, kinesthetic, and command.
- Associated with schizophrenia; postpartum psychosis; anorexia; depression with psychotic features; drug withdrawal; delirium; and bipolar, obsessive-compulsive, and body dysmorphic disorders.
- Recognize and accept that delusions and hallucinations are real and frightening to patient; stay with patient because isolation will increase hallucinations.
- Identify commands of violence that may harm self or others.
- Distract patient from delusions that may precipitate violence.
- Point out reality, but do not reason, argue, challenge patient.
- Focus on meaning and feelings rather than content.
- Praise reality-based perceptions.
- Identify factors that may exacerbate sensory and perceptual disturbances such as reflective glare, TV screens, and lights.
- Teach self-coping for delusions such as recreational and diversionary activities.
- Teach self-coping for hallucinations such as exercise, listening to music, saying "stop, go away!"; engage in structured activities.

Nursing Care for Patients With Dementia or Decreased Cognition

- Progressive disturbance in memory, speech, insight, judgment, reasoning, orientation; affect and behavior that interferes with ADLs; personality changes such as apathy or ↓ spontaneity and passivity *or* irritability, sarcasm, decreased concern for others, and/or self-preoccupation.

- Associated with vascular dementia and Alzheimer, Parkinson, Creutzfeldt-Jakob, and Pick diseases.
- Provide a safe, nonstimulating, familiar environment with consistent routines and caregiver.
- Use a calm, unhurried, nondemanding approach.
- Consider patient mood and easy distractibility when planning care.
- Reorient to time, place, person; use simple language and visual clues.
- Promote independence; assist with ADLs.
- Encourage reminiscing about earlier years.
- Identify events that increase agitation such as environmental stimuli, altered routines, strangers, increased expectations, "lost" items.
- Involve in simple, repetitive tasks and one-on-one activities.
- Promote involvement in therapy such as music, pet, and current events.
- Support primary caregivers and encourage periodic respite.

Nursing Care for Patients With Eating Disorders

- Preoccupation with weight involving ↓ or ↑ intake of food accompanied by weight loss behaviors such as purging, exercise, and abuse of laxatives or diuretics.
- Associated with anorexia and bulimia.
- Assist with contract for behavior-modification program such as eating and weight goals with consequences for goal attainment or failure.
- Observe for 1 hr after eating to prevent purging.
- Assess for fluid and electrolyte imbalances.
- Maintain matter-of-fact approach, shift focus from food, eating, and exercise to emotional issues.
- Provide and encourage intake of nutrient-dense foods.
- Support therapeutic interactions with individuals, groups, and family members.
- Identify issues of decreased self-esteem, identify disturbance, and family dysfunction.
- Provide ordered IV and/or tube feedings for patient with anorexia.

Nursing Care for Patients Who Are Hyperactive

- Increased motor activity and speech, impulsivity, inattention, and expansive and/or irritable mood.
- Associated with attention deficit hyperactivity disorder, bipolar disorder, manic and hypomanic episodes.

- Provide a safe, nonstimulating environment.
- Approach in a calm, nonargumentative manner.
- Channel hyperactivity into safe, controlled activities.
- Use easy distractibility to redirect inappropriate behavior.
- Keep activities simple, repetitive, and of short duration.
- Use rewards such as tokens and praise to reinforce appropriate behavior.
- Balance energy expenditure and rest.
- Provide high-protein, high-calorie, and handheld foods.

Nursing Care for Patients With Obsessive-Compulsive Disorder

- Uncontrollable desire to dwell on intrusive and inappropriate thoughts (**obsession**); repetitive actions to relieve anxiety connected with an obsession (**compulsion**).
- Associated with obsessive-compulsive disorders and anxiety.
- Know patient realizes the ritual is not rational but cannot control it.
- Allow performance of ritual until patient develops other defenses.
- Intervene when acting-out impulses may harm self or others.
- Limit time and frequency of ritual after other defenses develop.
- Reduce stress of decision making to decrease anxiety.
- Assist to identify and avoid anxiety-producing situations.
- Help to identify and use positive anxiety-reducing behaviors.

Nursing Care for Patients With Paranoia

- Suspicious thinking that is persecutory such as being harassed, poisoned, or judged critically.
- Associated with paranoid personality disorder, paranoid schizophrenia, and delusional paranoid disorder.
- Respect personal space; do not touch.
- Use nonthreatening body language; be calm and reassuring.
- Provide environment and activities that do not challenge security.
- Recognize and accept that delusions are real and frightening to patient.
- Identify presence of dangerous command hallucinations.
- Point out reality but do not directly challenge delusions.
- Praise reality-based perceptions.

Nursing Care for Patients With a Personality Disorder

- Persistent, pervasive, inflexible pattern of inner experience or behavior that deviates markedly from the norm.
  - **Cluster A**: Paranoid, schizoid, schizotypal.
  - **Cluster B**: Borderline, antisocial, histrionic, narcissistic.
  - **Cluster C**: Avoidant, dependent, obsessive-compulsive.
- Recognize development of trust will take time.
- Assess level of dependence and independence.
- Support decision making and independence.
- Involve patient in activities that ↑ self-esteem.
- Engage in social skills training specific to the disorder.
- Cluster A: See Nursing Care for Patients With Paranoia, p.167.
- Cluster B: See Nursing Care for Patients Who Are Hyperactive, p.166, and Nursing Care for Patients Who Are Aggressive, p.164.
- Cluster C: See Nursing Care for Patients Who Are Withdrawn, p.169, and Nursing Care for Patients With Obsessive-Compulsive Disorder, p.167.

Nursing Care for Patients Who Are Suicidal

- Increased risk for suicide is associated with mood disorders; command hallucinations; young adults and adolescents; single older adults; higher incidence with men; stress and loss; social isolation; substance abuse; hopelessness or helplessness; serious illness; sexual identity crisis; and physical or emotional abuse.
- **Levels of suicidal behavior**:
  - **Suicidal ideation**: Thoughts of suicide or self-injurious acts expressed verbally or symbolically.
  - **Suicide threat**: Expression of intent to commit suicide without action.
  - **Suicide gesture**: Self-directed act that results in minor injury.
  - **Suicidal attempt**: Self-directed act that may result in minor or major injury by person who intended to die.
  - **Suicide**: Self-inflicted death.
- Ask patient if there is a suicide plan, and identify if the patient has the means to carry it out.
- Encourage patient to write a no-suicide contract.
- Provide constant observation and safe environment such as no sharps, shoelaces, or cords; assign to a two-bedded room.
- Identify if patient is giving away possessions or putting affairs in order.
- Identify what precipitated or contributed to suicide crisis.
- Focus on patient's strengths rather than weaknesses.
- Encourage exploration of consequences if suicide attempt is unsuccessful, impact on others if successful, feelings about death, and reasons for living.

- Assist with problem solving; prioritize problems; focus on one at a time.
- Assist patient to write a list of support systems and community resources and how to ask for help.
- Ensure family members are aware of the need to maintain safety, as most suicides occur within 90 days after release from the hospital.

Nursing Care for Patients Who Are Withdrawn

- Patient retreats from people and reality.
- Associated with autism, depression, anxiety, schizophrenia, bipolar disorder depressive episode, avoidant and dependent personality disorders.
- Assess risk for suicide especially as depression and energy lift.
- Accept feelings of worthlessness as real.
- Sit quietly next to patient, then encourage one-on-one interaction.
- Spend time with patient to support worthiness; provide realistic praise.
- Accept but do not reward dependence; provide simple choices.
- Minimize isolation; involve in simple, repetitive activities.
- Assist to identify and replace self-deprecating thoughts with positive thoughts through cognitive restructuring.

Therapeutic Modalities

Nurse

- Therapeutic use of self to diagnose and treat human responses to actual or potential mental health problems.
- **Nursing care:** Engage in the activities such as health promotion; intake screening and evaluation; case management; support of self-care activities; psychobiological interventions; teaching; counseling; crisis intervention; milieu therapy; and psychosocial rehabilitation.

Individual Psychotherapy

- Patient and therapist enter into a therapeutic relationship.
- **Nursing care:** Assist to clarify perceptions; identify feelings; make connections among thoughts, feelings, and events; and increase insight.

Family Therapy

- Family treated as a unit; focuses on dynamics to attain and maintain balance and harmony.
- **Nursing care:** Help establish boundaries; assess hierarchy and subsystems; increase communication; increase interpersonal skills; and promote family cohesion and flexibility (see Group Therapy, below).

Milieu Therapy

- Therapeutic community; social structure is involved in helping process; interactions influence behavioral change.
- **Nursing care:** Provide clear communication; safe environment; activity schedule with therapeutic goals; and support network.

Self-Help Groups

- People have common beliefs, values, and behaviors.
- Must desire to change behavior; receive and give assistance to peers; leadership is shared by peers; lifelong process.
- **Nursing care:** Refer to appropriate group.

Behavioral Therapy

- Reward acceptable behaviors so they are reinforced (operant conditioning); based on fact that *behavior has consequences*; patients are active participants.
- **Nursing care:** Establish behavioral contract with goals and consequences; set firm, consistent limits on unacceptable behavior; and reward acceptable behavior and achievement of goals (token economy).

Group Therapy

- People share thoughts and feelings and help each other examine common issues and concerns.
- **Nursing care:** Refer to an appropriate group.

Stages of Group Process

Stage	Characteristics	Nursing Care
Beginning	Polite and congenial behavior initially; concerned with role and place in group; conflict dominates the end.	Provide orientation, set boundaries, help identify purpose and tasks.
Working	Develop rules, rituals, behavioral norms; develop cohesive, cooperative relationships; share ideas, experiences, feelings; focus on the present.	Provide structure, model acceptance, facilitate interaction, promote task accomplishment.
Termination	Begin to grieve for loss; attempt to reestablish self as individual.	Promote summary of group work, resist introduction of new topics, facilitate closure.

Psychoeducation

- Educational strategies to increase information and develop skills (**social skills training**); basis of psychosocial rehabilitation; individual or group.
- **Nursing care:**
  - Identify readiness to learn; begin at patient's level; build on strengths and experiences; individualize plan; give constructive feedback.
  - Perform demonstration and return demonstration; role-play.
  - Focus on information about etiology, treatment, stress management, and prognosis.
  - Develop communication, social, and problem-solving skills.

Light Therapy (Phototherapy)

- Exposure to bright full-spectrum fluorescent lamps suppresses melatonin production and normalizes disturbance in circadian rhythms; relieves depression of seasonal affective disorder (SAD); given from 30 min to 2–5 hr daily; depression begins to lift within 1–4 days; full effect in 2 weeks; maintained with daily sessions of 30 min.

- **Nursing care:**
  - Ensure ophthalmic consultation for preexisting eye problems; teach importance of arising before 8:00 a.m., sitting 3 feet from lights, engaging in other activities permitted but glancing at light every few minutes is necessary.
  - Assess for side effects such as eyestrain, headache, insomnia, and irritability.

Electroconvulsive Therapy (ECT)

- Short-acting barbiturate and muscle relaxant given before a brief electrical current is passed through brain to produce a generalized seizure; alters brain chemistry to improve mood; 2–3 treatments a week for 3–4 weeks.
- **Nursing care before ECT:** Witness informed consent; allay concerns and provide accurate information such as memory returns in 6–9 months and procedure is not painful; ensure ECG, physical exam, and lab work are done; no food and fluid after midnight; empty bladder; remove jewelry, dental appliances, and nail polish.
- **Nursing care during and after ECT:** Assess VS before, during, and after ECT; insert mouth guard; pre-oxygenate before and maintain oxygen after ECT; prevent harm during seizure; ensure patent airway after seizure; assess for side effects when patient awakens 10–15 min after ECT such as headache, muscle aches, confusion, and disorientation; usually disappears within 1 hr.

Seclusion and Restraint

- Place in single locked or unlocked safe room **(seclusion)**; physical restriction of movement **(restraint)**; protects patient and others from harm; standards are moving toward "no seclusion or restraint" policies.
- **Nursing care:**
  - Use less-restrictive interventions first; ensure restraint is not done for convenience, retaliation, coercion, or discipline.
  - When used in an emergency, a licensed independent primary health-care provider must perform face-to-face evaluation (1-hr rule); continuous in-person observation of patient for duration of use.
  - When seclusion only is used, audio and video equipment permitted after 1st hour; family must be notified.

Occupational Therapy

- Activities that increase attention span, motor/social skills, and ability with ADLs.

- **Nursing care:**
  - Function as a role model; encourage, support, teach, discuss, and promote reality testing of prescribed tasks.

Activity Therapy

- Therapeutic, expressive activity to ↓ pathology and ↑ mental and emotional health; ↑ awareness of feelings, behaviors, thoughts, and sensations.
- **Nursing care:**
  - Determine level of functioning; provide a variety of groups such as recreation, art, music, dance, movement, and pet therapy; support efforts.
  - Children benefit from play because they are less able to verbalize thoughts and feelings.
  - Patients with cognitive impairments do better in less challenging, low-functioning groups.

Crisis Intervention

- Assist to return to previous level of functioning; develop more constructive coping skills; short-term, goal-directed care.
- **Crisis:** A positive or negative sudden stressful experience perceived as threatening when usual coping does not maintain integrity; lasts from hours to a few weeks.
- **Phases:** Precipitating event; anxiety increases as coping becomes ineffective; internal and external resources are used to resolve the crisis; either resolution or panic with disorganization of the individual results.
- Influencing factors include individual's perception, personal coping mechanisms, and situational support.
- Types of crises:
  - **Maturational and developmental (internal):** Related to life events such as adolescence, completing school, marriage, childbirth, menopause and climacteric, retirement, and aging.
  - **Situational (external):** Related to unexpected situations such as relocation, loss of job, environmental disasters, and health problem.
  - **Adventitious:** Related to disasters such as floods, earthquakes, war, and terrorist attacks.
- **Nursing care:**
- Have patient describe event; support when confronting reality; encourage expression of feelings; clarify fantasies with facts.
- Explore strengths, weaknesses, and support systems.
- Assist with problem solving and developing new coping strategies; refer to community resources.

Psychopharmacology

- Drugs that affect emotion, behavior, and cognition include anxiolytics, mood stabilizers, stimulants, antidepressants, and antipsychotics.
- **Nursing care:** See Tab 7, MEDS, for sections addressing each of the drug classifications indicated above.

Neurological disorders
    Multiple Sclerosis
    Seizures
    Parkinson Disease
    Neurological Disorders With Respiratory Insufficiency
    Brain Attack (BA)/Cerebrovascular Accident (CVA)
    Spinal Cord Injury
Gastrointestinal Disorders
    Morbid Obesity
    Gastroesophageal Reflux Disease (GERD) and Hiatal Hernia
    Peptic Ulcer Disease and Gastric Carcinoma
    Lower GI Disorders
Disorders of Accessory Organs of Digestion
    Cholecystitis
    Hepatitis
    Cirrhosis
    Pancreatitis
Nursing Care for Patients Receiving Nutritional Support
    Parenteral Nutrition (PN)
    Enteral Nutrition (Tube Feeding)
Female Reproductive Cancers
    Breast Cancer
    Cervical Cancer
    Ovarian Cancer
Infectious Diseases
    Lyme Disease and Tetanus
    HIV and AIDS
Perioperative Nursing Care
    Preoperative Nursing Care
    Intraoperative Nursing Care
    Postoperative Nursing Care

Care of Patients With Cancer

Cancer (Ca) is the mutation of cellular DNA resulting in abnormal cells that invade other tissue by extension or metastasis via lymph or blood.

Types

Adenocarcinoma (glandular), carcinoma (epithelial), glioma (central nervous system [CNS]), leukemia (blood forming), lymphoma (lymphatic), melanoma (pigmented), myeloma (plasma of bone marrow), sarcoma (soft tissue, muscle, vascular, synovial).

Risk Factors

Genetics, microbiological agents (herpes simplex virus/cervical Ca), physical agents (sun exposure/skin Ca), hormones (estrogen/breast Ca), chemical agents (smoking/lung Ca), diet ($\uparrow$ fat/colon Ca), $\downarrow$ immune response (AIDS/Kaposi sarcoma).

Early Detection

■ See BASICS, Tab 1, CAUTION, p. 19.
■ Screening: Yearly cervical Pap tests at 18 yr; yearly clinical breast exam and monthly self breast exam (SBE) at 20 yr; yearly mammogram at 40 yr; yearly fecal occult blood test at 50 yr; colonoscopy every 5–10 yr at 50 yr; and digital rectal exam for prostate changes at 50 yr.

Staging

Staging helps determine treatment and prognosis; see TNM Staging.

TNM Staging

Size of Tumor (T)	Nodal Involvement (N)	Metastasis (M)
TX: Not assessable. TO: No evidence of tumor. Tis: In situ. T1–4: Increasing tumor size.	NX: Not assessable. NO: No metastasis to regional nodes. N1–3: Increasing regional node involvement.	MX: Not assessable. MO: No metastasis. M1: Metastasis.

General Nursing Care for Patients With Cancer

■ Teach healthy lifestyle (no smoking, weight control, $\downarrow$ fat diet with $\uparrow$ intake of cruciferous vegetables and carotenoids, $\downarrow$ sun exposure).
■ Encourage routine screening; refer to American Cancer Society.
■ Support pain management.
■ Support advanced directives (living will, health-care proxy), decision for palliative/hospice care.
■ Document patient status and nursing interventions; notify health-care provider if infection, bleeding, fluid and electrolyte (F&E) imbalances, tumor lysis syndrome, nephrotoxicity, hepatotoxicity, or cardiotoxicity occur.

Nursing Care for Patients With Cancer or Experiencing Nontherapeutic Effects of Antineoplastic Therapies

Anorexia
- Obtain a calorie count, weigh weekly.
- Plan small frequent, bland meals; support food preferences.
- Increase protein and calories, provide supplements between meals.

Nausea and Vomiting (N&V)
- Assess for signs and symptoms (S&S) of F&E imbalances; monitor intake and output (I&O).
- Prevent aspiration.
- Provide adequate hydration.
- Hold food and fluids 4–6 hr before chemotherapy that causes N&V.
- Give prescribed antiemetic, usually via IV 30–45 min before and for 24 hr after caustic med.

Inflammation of Oral Mucosa (Stomatitis)
- Assess mucous membranes, gag reflex, ability to chew or swallow.
- Avoid extreme temperatures of food/fluid and spicy foods/fluids.
- Provide ordered puree/fluid diet.
- Rinse mouth with normal saline every 2 hr; provide popsicles for moisture.
- Use sponge toothbrush, avoid mouthwash, remove dentures except when eating.
- Give prescribed topical antiseptics/analgesics (swish and spit, or swish and swallow).

Rectal Sores or Bleeding
- Assess for occult or frank blood in stool.
- Apply prescribed topical ointments/warm compresses to rectum.
- Avoid suppositories and taking rectal temps.

Alopecia
- Assess self-esteem, provide emotional support.
- Explain that hair eventually will grow back but may be a different color/texture.
- Use mild shampoo and wide-tooth comb, minimize combing, avoid hair dryers and curling irons, wear hat in sun.
- Encourage purchase of a wig and cutting hair before hair loss.

Diarrhea
- Assess perianal skin; S&S of F&E imbalances.
- Provide perianal skin care; use barrier ointment.
- Give prescribed antidiarrheals.

Fatigue
- Assess activity tolerance.
- Balance activity/rest; organize activities to provide uninterrupted rest.
- Encourage delegation of responsibilities to conserve energy.

Decreased Platelets (Thrombocytopenia)
- Assess for S&S of bleeding: Ecchymosis, petechiae, hematuria, melena, hematemesis, hemoptysis, bleeding from gums or venipuncture sites, ↓ platelets, ↓ hematocrit (Hct), ↓ hemoglobin (Hb).
- Avoid taking rectal temps, use electric razor, use emery board for nail care.
- Use smallest gauge needle for injections, compress venipuncture site for 5–10 min.
- Avoid aspirin, NSAIDs, alcohol.
- Administer ordered platelets.

Decreased Leukocytes (↓ White Blood Cells [WBCs], Neutropenia)
- Assess for S&S of infection (↑ temperature [T], chills, diaphoresis); monitor WBCs count.
- Provide neutropenic precautions when WBCs ≤1000/mm³: Private room; eliminate fresh fruits, vegetables, flowers/potted plants; avoid people with infections.
- Obtain specimen for culture and sensitivity (C&S) before initiating prescribed antibiotic.
- Provide care for sites of potential microbial growth (IV and catheter sites, wounds, skin folds, perineum, oral cavity).
- Give prescribed medications to ↑WBCs such as filgrastim (Neupogen), pegfilgrastim (Neulasta).

Decreased Red Blood Cells (RBCs)
- Monitor RBCs, Hb, Hct.
- Assess for tachycardia, pallor, fatigue; encourage rest.
- Give prescribed epoetin (Epogen) and blood products (packed red blood cells [PRBCs]) to ↑ RBCs.

Nephrotoxicity
- Monitor blood urea nitrogen (BUN), creatinine, creatinine clearance, F&E, I&O.
- Provide 2–3 L of fluid daily.
- Assess for S&S of gout; give prescribed allopurinol (Zyloprim) to prevent uric acid crystals.

Cardiotoxicity
- Assess for dyspnea, crackles, ↑ respiration (R), peripheral edema, ↑ weight.
- Assess for tachycardia, dysrhythmias.

Hepatotoxicity
- Assess for N&V, malaise, bruising, bleeding, jaundice.
- Monitor liver function test results.

Tissue Necrosis From Extravasation of a Vesicant
- Ensure IV is in vein and patent.
- Assess for infiltration or inflammation of IV site.
- Discontinue (D/C), restart in another vein if indicated; elevate extremity for 24 hr; apply ice or warm compresses as per protocol.

Tumor Lysis Syndrome
- Assess for hyperkalemia, hypocalcemia, hyperphosphatemia, hyperuricemia (destroyed tumor cells release excessive intracellular metabolites).
- Administer prescribed IV fluids, sodium polystyrene sulfonate (Kayexalate), allopurinol (Zyloprim), phosphate-binding gels.

Renal and Urinary Tract Disorders

Urinary Tract Infections (UTIs)

Lower UTI: Urethritis, Cystitis
Ascending pathogens such as *E. coli* cause inflammation of the urethra (urethritis) and inflammation of the bladder (cystitis); may lead to bacterial sepsis and kidney failure.

Risk Factors
- Catheterization, female gender, incontinence, ↑ age, diabetes mellitus (DM).

Signs and Symptoms
- Frequency, urgency, burning.
- Bacteria, RBCs, and WBCs in urine; ↑ serum WBCs.

Treatment
- Urine and blood cultures as needed (prn).
- Antibiotics, antispasmodics, urinary tract antiseptics, sulfonamides, urinary tract analgesic such as phenazopyridine (Pyridium).
- Sepsis requires IV fluid replacement, antibiotics, nutritional support.

Nursing Care
- Assess for S&S, C&S to determine appropriateness of antibiotic, ↑ fluids to 3–4 L daily, encourage patient to empty bladder every 3–4 hr, provide perineal care.
- Maintain indwelling catheter: Surgical asepsis during insertion, closed system, secure to leg to prevent movement in and out of urethra, keep collection bag lower than bladder.

Upper UTI: Pyelonephritis

Urine reflux from bladder into ureters (**ureterovesical reflux**) or obstruction causes inflammation of the renal pelvis; may lead to bacterial sepsis and kidney failure.

Risk Factors
■ Calculi, stricture, enlarged prostate, incompetent ureterovesical valve.

Signs and Symptoms
■ ↑T, chills, N&V.
■ Tender costovertebral angle (**flank pain**).

Treatment and Nursing Care
■ See Treatment and Nursing Care under Lower UTI, p. 180.

Upper UTI: Glomerulonephritis

Infections elsewhere in the body precipitate inflammation of glomerular capillaries; may lead to bacterial sepsis and kidney failure.

Risk Factors
■ Beta-hemolytic streptococcal throat infection.
■ Bacterial, viral, or parasitic infection elsewhere in the body.
■ Exogenous antigens such as medications.

Signs and Symptoms
■ Hematuria, proteinuria, ↓ urination.

Treatment and Nursing Care
■ See Treatment and Nursing Care under Lower UTI, p. 180.

Prostate Disorders: Benign Prostatic Hyperplasia (BPH) and Prostate Cancer

BPH

Enlarged prostate → urethral constriction → urinary retention → ↑ risk for UTI, hydronephrosis, and hydroureter.

Prostate Cancer

Cancerous cells in prostate; may metastasize to pelvis, bone, lymph nodes, liver.

Risk Factors
■ ↑ age, familial history, African heritage, ↑ intake of red meat, smoking.

Signs and Symptoms
- Frequency, urgency, ↓ stream, hesitancy, nocturia, retention, sexual dysfunction.
- *Prostate cancer:* Prostatic-specific antigen (PSA) >2 ng/mL; confirmed by biopsy.
- *Bony metastasis:* Back/hip pain, ↓ weight, fatigue, anemia, ↑ alkaline phosphatase.

Treatment
- *BPH:* Alpha blockers (terazosin [Hytrin]), antiandrogens (finasteride), heat, lasers, surgery (transurethral resection [TUR]; suprapubic prostatectomy).
- *Cancer:* Radical prostatectomy, orchiectomy, radiation, hormonal therapy (estrogen).

Nursing Care
- Assess for S&S; provide indwelling catheter care; give prescribed medications.
- Provide postoperative care:
  - Traction on catheter balloon if present to ↓ bleeding
  - Continuous bladder irrigation (CBI): Three-way catheter to maintain patency.
  - Discuss concerns about sexual dysfunction, urine dribbling.

Urolithiasis (Kidney Stones, Calculi)

- Urinary stasis or chemical environment that → precipitation and crystallization of minerals; stones form that obstruct the ureter, resulting in hydroureter and hydronephrosis; stones can recur.
- Components of calculi vary: Calcium with phosphorus or oxalate (75%); uric acid (10%); struvite (15%); cystine (1%).

Risk Factors
- 30–50 yr, male, dehydration, diet with ↑ dairy and vitamin D.
- ↑ UTIs (struvite calculi), hyperparathyroidism (calcium calculi), gout and myeloprolific disease increase uric acid (uric acid calculi).

Signs and Symptoms
- Pain, depending on stone location; may have little or no pain ranging to severe pain radiating from flank to bladder or genitals.
- N&V, hematuria, pallor, diaphoresis, UTI.

Treatment
- Opioids, NSAIDs.
- Calcium stones: Ammonium chloride to acidify urine, thiazide diuretics.
- Uric acid stones: Allopurinol (Zyloprim), ↑ urine pH.

- Lithotripsy: Extracorporeal shock wave, percutaneous ultrasonic, or laser.
- Diet based on stone composition, hydration.

Nursing Care
- Assess for S&S, strain urine, ↑ fluids to 3–4 L daily, control pain.
- Calcium stones: Acid ash diet with ↓ dairy, protein, and Na intake.
- Uric acid stones: Alkaline ash diet with ↓ purine (organ meat) intake.
- Oxalate stones: ↓ tea, spinach, nuts, chocolate, and rhubarb intake.

Kidney Failure

Acute Kidney Failure	End Stage Renal Disease (ESRD)
• ↓ glomerular filtration rate due to ↓ kidney perfusion, tubular or glomeruli damage, obstruction. • Moves from <100 mL **(anuria)** or <400 mL **(oliguria)** to ↑ urine output **(diuresis)**. • Progresses to recovery or ESRD. • **Risk factors:** Hemorrhage; septic shock; ↓ cardiac output; myoglobinuria due to burns or crushing injury; nephrotoxic agents; transfusion reaction; calculi; BPH; infections.	• Progressive, irreversible ↓ nephron function → uremia, retention of water, potassium, and phosphorus. • Metabolic acidosis due to inability to excrete ammonia and reabsorb bicarbonate. • **Risk factors:** DM; ↑ blood pressure (BP); chronic infections (pyelonephritis, glomerulonephritis); polycystic kidney disease; nephrotoxic agents (amino-glycosides, lead, mercury, NSAIDs).

Signs and Symptoms
- ↓ urine output, ↑ BUN, ↑ creatinine, ↑ K, ↑ phosphate, ↓ calcium.
- *Metabolic acidosis:* ↓ pH, ↓ HCO_3, ↓ CO_2, ↑ BP, Kussmaul respirations, pro-teinuria, lethargy, confusion, headache, seizures, nausea, anemia due to ↓ erythropoietin, fluid excess (dyspnea, crackles, ↑ P, ↑ R, distended neck veins).

Treatment
- Epoetin alfa (Epogen, Procrit), calcium carbonate, antihypertensives.
- ↓ fluid, sodium (Na), potassium intake; ↓ dietary protein to ↓ nitrogenous wastes.
- Hemo- or peritoneal dialysis; hemofiltration.
- ESRD: Renal transplant with immunosuppressives to prevent rejection.

Nursing Care

- Assess for S&S and adherence to diet; weigh before and after dialysis.
- *Hemodialysis:* Assess patency of graft/fistula if present (auscultate bruit, palpate thrill); avoid trauma to arm (no injections, IV, BP).
- *Assess for complications of hemodialysis:* ↓ BP, air embolism, dysrhythmias, atherosclerosis.
- *Peritoneal dialysis:* Instill and drain dialysate via gravity, assess for dyspnea (if present may need to drain fluid), periodically alternate patient position.
- *Assess for complications of peritoneal dialysis:* Peritonitis, ↑ triglycerides, dyspnea and hernias due to ↑ abdominal pressure.
- *Kidney transplant:* Explain need for lifelong immunosuppressive drugs → ↑ infection.
- *Assess for S&S of rejection:* Oliguria, ↑T, ↑ creatinine, flank pain.

Fluid, Electrolyte, and Acid-Base Disturbances

Common Imbalances: Fluids and Potassium

Fluid Deficit	Fluid Excess
• **Hypovolemia:** Proportional loss of extracellular fluid (ECF) volume and electrolytes.	• **Hypervolemia:** ↑ ECF volume.
• **Dehydration:** Loss of only water with ↑ Na related to following causes.	• **Causes:** Heart or renal failure, cirrhosis, ↑ Na, excess IV fluids, ↓ albumin, ↑ aldosterone secretion.
• **Causes:** N&V, diarrhea, GI suction, sweating, ↓ fluid intake, diuretics, adrenal insufficiency.	• **Syndrome of inappropriate antidiuretic hormone (SIADH):** ↑ ADH → water retention and ↓ Na due to disorders of CNS and lungs, infections, malignant tumors.
• **S&S:** ↓ weight, ↓ turgor, dry skin, muscle weakness/cramps, thirst, oliguria, postural hypotension, ↑T, ↑ P, ↑ Hct, ↑ BUN, ↑ specific gravity.	• **S&S:** ↑T, ↑ P, ↑ BP, edema, ascites, crackles, jugular vein distention, ↓ Hct, ↓ BUN.
• **Nursing Care:** Assess for S&S; ↑ oral fluids; give prescribed isotonic/hypotonic IV fluids, prescribed prn antiemetics or antidiarrheals.	• **Nursing Care:** Assess for S&S; teach ↓ Na diet, fluid restriction, Na content of over-the-counter (OTC) meds; give prescribed diuretics and potassium supplements.

Hypokalemia	Hyperkalemia
• Potassium (K) <3.5 mEq/L.	• Potassium (K) >5 mEq/L.
• **Causes:** Vomiting; diarrhea; gastric suction; diuretics; corticosteroids; diabetic ketoacidosis **(osmotic diuresis)**; starvation; if taking digoxin, hypokalemia → ↑ risk of digoxin toxicity.	• **Causes:** Kidney disease, burns, crushing injury, metabolic acidosis, adrenal insufficiency, excess K supplements.
• **S&S:** Muscle weakness, fatigue, N&V, ↓ GI motility, ↓ reflexes, abdominal distention, dysrhythmias, elevated U wave and flattened T wave on ECG.	• **S&S:** Dysrhythmias; peaked T waves, flattened P waves, and wide QRS complexes on ECG; muscle weakness; flaccid paralysis; intestinal colic; diarrhea.
• **Nursing Care:** Assess for S&S, teach about foods high in K (melon, apricots, bananas, milk, meat, citrus, grains).	• **Nursing Care:** Assess for S&S; avoid salt substitutes and K-sparing diuretics with renal disease.
• **Meds:** Give ordered IV or oral K supplements.	• **Meds:** Give prescribed calcium gluconate IV; regular insulin with glucose; sodium bicarbonate; exchange resin (Kayexalate).

Common Imbalances: Sodium and Calcium

Hyponatremia	Hypernatremia
• Sodium (Na) <135 mEq/L.	• Sodium (Na) >145 mEq/L.
• **Causes:** Vomiting, diarrhea, gastric suction, sweating, excess intake of Na-free fluids, diuretics, renal disease, adrenal insufficiency, SIADH.	• **Causes:** Diarrhea, ↓ fluid intake, heat stroke, excess Na intake (near drowning in ocean, sodium bicarbonate, hypertonic NaCl).
• **S&S:** Muscle cramps; weakness; papilledema, headache, confusion, seizures due to ↑ intracranial pressure (ICP).	• **S&S:** Thirst; ↑ T; ↑ P; ↑ BP; dry, sticky mucous membranes; N&V; ↑ reflexes; restlessness; seizures.
• **Nursing Care:** Assess for S&S, ↑ Na intake, give IVF (usually normal saline), ↓ fluids to 800 mL/daily as ordered.	• **Nursing Care:** Assess for S&S; give ordered IVF (D$_5$W, hypotonic solution) and prescribed diuretics.

Continued

Hypocalcemia	Hypercalcemia
• Calcium (Ca) <8.5 mEq/L.	• Calcium (Ca) >10.5 mEq/L.
• **Causes:** Hypoparathyroidism, renal failure, malabsorption, ↓ albumin, ↓ vitamin D, alkalosis, pancreatitis, meds (loop diuretics, steroids, some antineoplastics, isoniazid [INH]).	• **Causes:** Immobility, bone cancer, hyperparathyroidism, meds (thiazide diuretics, lithium, excess calcium or vitamin D supplements).
• **S&S:** Paresthesias, tetany, facial nerve twitching (**Chvostek sign**), carpopedal spasm (**Trousseau sign**), ↑ ST segment on ECG; confusion, seizures.	• **S&S:** Deep bone pain, flank pain due to renal calculi, constipation, vomiting, ↓ reflexes, ↑ urine calcium (**Sulkowitch test**), osteoporosis, ↑ hyperparathyroid hormone (PTH) levels, ↓ PTH levels (with malignancy).
• **Nursing Care:** Assess for S&S; give prescribed calcium and vitamin D supplements; teach high-calcium foods (milk, salmon, green leafy vegetables, sardines).	• **Nursing Care:** Assess for S&S; ↑ fluids; ↑ fiber; give prescribed IVF and meds (calcitonin, loop diuretic, bisphosphonate).

Common Imbalances: Acid-Base

Metabolic Acidosis	Metabolic Alkalosis
• Serum pH <7.35 and bicarbonate (HCO_3) <22 mEq/L.	• Serum pH >7.45 and bicarbonate (HCO_3) >26 mEq/L.
• **Causes:** ↑ acid (ASA poisoning, lactic or ketoacidosis, uremia); ↓ HCO_3 (diarrhea, chlorides, diuretics); hypoproteinemia.	• **Causes:** Loss of acidic gastric secretions (vomiting, gastric suction), thiazide and loop diuretics, ↑ intake of sodium bicarbonate.
• **S&S:** Headache, confusion, weakness, fruity breath, ↑ rate and ↑ depth of respirations (**Kussmaul respirations**), N&V, dysrhythmias, coma.	• **S&S:** Paresthesias, muscle hypertonicity, tremors, ↓ rate and ↓ depth of respirations, dizziness, confusion, coma.
• **Nursing Care:** Assess for S&S, give prescribed sodium bicarbonate, supportive care for underlying problem.	• **Nursing Care:** Assess for S&S; give prescribed NaCl fluids, KCl replacement, and H_2 antagonists.

Respiratory Acidosis	Respiratory Alkalosis
• Serum pH <7.35 and $Paco_2$ >45 mm Hg. • **Causes:** ↓ ventilation and CO_2 retention from pulmonary edema, pneumonia, acute respiratory distress syndrome (ARDS), narcotic overdose, aspiration, emphysema, obstructed airway, neuromuscular disease, apnea. • **S&S:** Shortness of breath (SOB), ↑ P, ↑ R, ↑ BP, restlessness, disorientation, cyanosis, coma. • **Nursing Care:** Assess for S&S; care for underlying cause (antibiotics, bronchodilators, thrombolytics); ↑ oxygenation (suction airway, Fowler position, mechanical ventilation).	• Serum pH >7.45 and $Paco_2$ <35 mm Hg. • **Causes:** Blowing off CO_2 due to hyperventilation or excess mechanical ventilation. • **S&S:** Deep, rapid breathing; ↑ P; paresthesias; light-headedness; dysrhythmias; ↓ level of consciousness (LOC). • **Nursing Care:** Assess for S&S; teach to breathe slowly or breathe into a paper bag; give prescribed sedative; ↓ rate and/or depth of ventilator settings as ordered.

Integumentary Disorders

Burns

Thermal, electrical, or chemical trauma → tissue destruction; intensity and duration of heat determine depth of destruction; prognosis depends on location and % of total body surface area (TBSA) involved.

Extent of Burn
- *Rule of nines:* Body divided into sections by % to quickly assess TBSA involved; head and neck (9%), each arm (9%), anterior trunk (18%), posterior trunk (18%), each leg (18%), perineum (1%).
  - *Minor:* <15% TBSA; face, hands, feet, and genitals not involved.
  - *Moderate:* Partial thickness 15%–25% or full thickness <10%.
  - *Major:* Partial thickness >25%; full thickness >10%; burns of face, hands, feet, or genitals, other complications.

Depth of burn
- *Partial-thickness (superficial):* Includes epidermis; may include top layer of dermis; erythema; pain; blanching with pressure.
- *Partial-thickness (deep):* Includes deeper layer of dermis; erythema; hypersensitive to touch/air; moderate to severe pain; moist blebs; blisters.

- *Full-thickness:* Extends through dermis and may involve underlying tissue; pale, white, or brown charred appearance **(eschar)**; edema; absence of pain in burned tissue but severe pain in surrounding tissue; burn odor.
- *Inhalation injury:* Facial burns, singed nostril hair, sooty sputum, voice change, blisters in mouth or throat, dyspnea.

Burn Phases

- *Emergent or immediate resuscitative phase:* Onset of injury to 5 or more days; usually 24–48 hr; from fluid loss and edema formation until diuresis begins.
- *Acute phase:* Weeks or months; from mobilization of extracellular fluid to diuresis; burned area is covered by skin grafts or until wounds heal.
- *Rehabilitation phase:* 2 weeks to 2–3 months; major wound closure to achievement of maximal physical and psychosocial adjustment; mature healing of skin may take 6 months–2 yr.

Signs and Symptoms

- *Emergent or immediate resuscitative phase:* Shock from pain and hypovolemia; fluid shift to interstitial and third spaces; edema; adynamic ileus; shivering related to heat loss, anxiety, pain; altered mental state (hypoxia due to smoke inhalation, pain medications); ↑ Hct; impairment of immune system (↓ WBCs).
- *Acute phase:* ↓ edema; necrotic tissue sloughs; granulation occurs in partial-thickness burns (10–14 days).
- *Rehabilitation phase:* Flat, pink new skin becomes raised and hyperemic in 4–6 weeks and will cause joint flexion and fixation **(contracture)** if not prevented; altered contour (slightly elevated and enlarged over burn injury) minimized with pressure; pain replaced by itchiness.

Treatment

At Scene of Burn

- Extinguishing of flames.
- Maintenance of airway, breathing, circulation.
- First aid to prevent shock and respiratory distress.
- Application of cool water briefly to ↓ trauma and pain (avoid ice because it ↑ damage); rapid sustained flushing of skin/eyes if chemical burn.
- Removal of clothing and jewelry to prevent constriction as edema progresses; leave adherent clothing.
- Burn covered with sterile/clean dressing (no ointments).

In Hospital

- May require intubation, oxygen, mechanical ventilation.
- Assessment of extent and depth of burns; hemodynamic monitoring; ECG for electrical burns.

- Fluid replacement using an established formula (1/2 of fluids in first 8 hr and other 1/2 over next 16 hr).
- Prevention of electrolyte imbalance (hyper/hypokalemia and hyper/hyponatremia).
- IV opioids to ↓ pain; antisecretories to prevent Curling ulcer; tetanus toxoid; topical and systemic antibiotics.
- Wound care; pressure garments to ↓ scars, splints to ↓ contractures.
- ↑ calorie and protein intake; vitamins and iron.

During Rehabilitation
- Physical therapy (PT), occupational therapy (OT), vocational education.
- Reconstruction (cosmetic, functional).
- Counseling to manage ↓ function, disfigurement, economic burden, and return to work.

Nursing Care

Emergent or Immediate Resuscitative Phase
- Maintain respirations and patent airway (suction, endotracheal tube, mechanical ventilator); place in Fowler position.
- Assess arterial blood gases (ABGs), oxygen saturation, breath sounds.
- Assess fluid shift from intravascular to interstitial space.
- Assess hourly urine output and for S&S of hyperkalemia.
- Encourage coughing and deep breathing; teach use of incentive spirometer.

Acute Phase
- Assess fluid shift from interstitial to intravascular space; assess for S&S of hypokalemia.

Rehabilitation Phase
- Continue assessing for infection and providing nutritional support until skin coverage is achieved.
- Protect new skin from injury; teach self-care and wound care.
- Reassure appearance will continue to improve over time; refer to support group.

All Phases
- *Maintain fluid balance:* Assess for S&S of fluid shifts and edema; monitor daily weight, I&O, hemodynamic status; give ordered oral fluids.
- *Maintain circulation:* Provide ordered IV F&E and colloids; ensure urinary output ≥30–50 mL/hr; systolic BP ≥100 mm Hg, and P ≤120 bpm.
- *Prevent infection:* Assess for S&S of infection (↑T, ↑WBCs, wound bed and donor sites for purulent drainage, edema, and redness); use contact precautions; give prescribed systemic/topical antimicrobials/antibiotics; provide ordered surgical aseptic wound care.

- *Manage pain:* Give pain medications before procedures and routinely before pain increases; use nonpharmacological interventions such as distraction, imagery; use lifting sheet; keep room temperature 80–85°F, humidity >40%; prevent drafts.
- *Maintain nutrition:* Nothing by mouth (NPO) initially; tube feedings or parenteral nutrition; high-calorie, high-protein diet with supplements when ordered.
- *Provide emotional support:* Address fear, grief, altered role, body image; explain that edema will subside in 2–4 days; explain all care.
- *Maintain bowel function:* Nasogastric tube (NGT) to decompression (↓ N&V, aspiration, ileus formation); assess bowel function (bowel sounds, stool).
- *Ongoing care:* Assist with hydrotherapy, débridement, grafting; plan for rest; maintain mobility and prevent contractures (positioning, splints, ambulation, range of motion [ROM]); teach use of pressure garments and skin lubrication; ↑ self-care activities when able.

Hormonal Disorders

Addison Disease

- Adrenocortical disorder exhibited by ↓ secretion of adrenocortical hormones (glucocorticoids, mineralocorticoids [aldosterone], and androgens), which → ↓ stress response.
- Causes: Surgical removal of adrenal glands, autoimmune or idiopathic causes, abrupt cessation of steroid therapy, infection.

Signs and Symptoms
- Dehydration, ↓ serum glucose, weakness, diarrhea, confusion, ↓ BP, ↓ weight, bronze-colored skin.
- ↑ adrenocorticotropic hormone (ACTH), ↓ serum cortisol, ↓ 17-ketosteroids, ↓ 17-hydroxysteroids, ↑ K, ↓ Na.
- *Addisonian crisis:* Pallor or cyanosis, anxiety, ↑ P, ↑ R, ↓ BP due to acute stress (surgery, emotions, cold exposure, infection).

Treatment
- Glucocorticoid and mineralocorticoid replacement (↑ dose under stress to ↓ risk of Addisonian crisis).
- F&E replacement.

Nursing Care
- Assess for S&S of Addisonian crisis.
- Encourage ↑ protein and ↑ carbohydrate diet with added salt.
- Teach need for lifelong therapy, avoidance of stress, balance of rest and exercise, and use of medical alert band.

Cushing Syndrome

- Adrenocortical disorder exhibited by ↑ secretion of adrenocortical hormones (glucocorticoids, mineralocorticoids [aldosterone], and androgens), which → ↓ immune response; ↑ Na; water retention; ↑ serum glucose.
- Causes: Adrenal tumor, or ↑ ACTH from pituitary, steroid therapy.

Signs and Symptoms

- Truncal obesity, thin extremities due to muscle wasting, buffalo hump and moon face due to fluid retention, acne, hirsutism, purple abdominal striae, ↓ libido, S&S of hypervolemia.
- ↑ serum cortisol, ↑ 17-ketosteroids, ↑ 17-hydroxysteroids, ↓ K, ↑ Na, ↓ ACTH (↑ ACTH if due to a pituitary problem), ↑ glucose.
- ↑ risk of infection, osteoporosis, psychosis.

Treatment

- Adrenalectomy or removal of pituitary tumor (**hypophysectomy**), depending on cause.
- Adrenal enzyme inhibitors: Aminoglutethimide, mitotane.
- If resulting from steroid therapy, reduce steroids slowly.
- Treat complications such as DM, osteoporosis.

Nursing Care

- Assess for S&S.
- Encourage ↓ Na and ↑ K in diet as ordered.
- Protect from infection and injury because of ↑ risk for fractures due to osteoporosis.
- Encourage use of medical alert band.
- Provide emotional support for altered body image and labile mood.

Diabetes Mellitus (DM)

- *Normal glucose metabolism:* Blood glucose regulated by the hormones insulin and glucagon; glucose is stored as glycogen in liver and muscles or as fat in adipose tissue.
- *Action of insulin:* Secreted by beta cells in islets of Langerhans in pancreas; insulin decreases blood glucose by promoting its entry into cells.
- *Action of glucagon:* Secreted by alpha cells in pancreas as blood glucose falls; promotes release of glycogen from liver.
- *DM:* Decreased amount of insulin or ↓ response to insulin leads to ↑ blood glucose (**hyperglycemia**).

Type 1

- 10% of DM; beta cell destruction → little or no insulin for cellular metabolism of glucose; requires exogenous insulin.
- Associated with specific human leukocyte antigens (HLA); autoantibodies; viruses; presents at <30 yr of age.

Type 2

- 90% of DM; ↓ sensitivity to insulin (**insulin resistance**) and ↓ secretion of insulin; may be controlled by diet, exercise, and hypoglycemics; may need insulin when stressed.
- Associated with obesity, genetics, inactivity, gestational diabetes; usually presents at >45 yr of age; increasing incidence in children.

Signs and Symptoms

- *The 3 Ps:* **P**olyuria, **P**olydipsia, **P**olyphagia (excessive urination, thirst, hunger).
- Fasting blood glucose >126 mg/dL, random blood glucose >200 mg/dL.
- >7% glycated hemoglobin (hemoglobin A_{1C}) indicates lack of glucose control over prior 3 months; glycosuria.
- Risk for infection; ↓ healing; type 1 –↓ weight; type 2—↑ weight.
- Long-term complications:
  - *Microvascular changes:* Retinopathy, neuropathy, nephropathy.
  - *Macrovascular changes:* Peripheral vascular disease (PVD), ischemic heart disease, cerebral vascular disease.

Alterations in Blood Glucose Associated With DM

Hyperglycemia	Hypoglycemia
• Blood glucose >110 mg/dL (>6.1 mmol/L). • **Causes:** Stress, omission of hypoglycemic med or insulin, excess food intake; develops over days. • **S&S:** Polyuria; thirst; dry, hot, red skin; blurred vision; confusion; ↑ P; ↓ BP; S&S of dehydration.	• Blood glucose <60 mg/dL (<2.7 mmol/L). • **Causes:** Excess insulin or oral diabetic meds; ↑ exercise or ↓ food while taking antidiabetic meds; develops rapidly. • **S&S:** Nervousness; pallor; cool, clammy skin; ↑ P; tremors; slurred speech; seizure.

Alterations in Blood Glucose Associated With DM—cont'd

Hyperglycemic Hyperosmolar Nonketotic Syndrome (HHNS)	Diabetic Ketoacidosis (DKA)
• Serum glucose >600 mg/dL without ketonuria; associated with type 2 DM. • **Causes:** Stress (surgery, infection), ↓ hypoglycemic meds, ↑ food intake. • **S&S:** S&S of hyperglycemia, no ketones in urine, no S&S of metabolic acidosis.	• Serum glucose >300–600 mg/dL; breakdown of fat to meet energy needs causes ketonuria; associated with type 1 DM. • **Causes:** Stress (surgery, infection); ↓ exogenous insulin; ↑ food intake; meds such as steroids. • **S&S:** S&S of hyperglycemia, ketonuria; S&S of metabolic acidosis.
Somogyi Effect	**Dawn Phenomenon**
• Hypoglycemia ↑ release of epinephrine, corticosteroids, and growth hormone, causing rebound hyperglycemia; hyperglycemia at hours of sleep (hs) with hypoglycemia at 2 a.m. followed by rebound hyperglycemia in morning.	• Marked increase in insulin requirements between 6–9 a.m. compared to midnight to 6 a.m.

Treatment

■ Regular exercise to control weight and ↓ insulin resistance.
■ Balance diet (50%–60% carbohydrates, 20% protein, 20%–30% fat) based on glycemic food index; ↑ soluble fiber → slow glucose absorption.
■ Insulin and/or oral hypoglycemics.
■ Pancreatic or islets of Langerhans transplants.
■ *DKA and HHNS:* IVF, rapid or short-acting insulin, eventual Na and K replacement.
■ *Hypoglycemia:* 10–15 g of simple sugar followed by complex carbohydrate and protein if conscious; glucagon injection or 50% dextrose IV if unconscious.
■ *Somogyi effect:* Requires increased insulin adjustment.
■ *Dawn phenomenon:* Requires decreased insulin adjustment.

Nursing Care

- *Assess for S&S of alterations in blood glucose:* Hyperglycemia, hypoglycemia, DKN, HHNS, Somogyi effect, and dawn phenomenon.
- Provide foot care:
  - Inspect daily for lesions.
  - Wash/dry between toes daily, wear socks and well-fitting shoes, avoid heat/cold.
- Encourage weight-control efforts and continued health-care supervision (certified diabetic educator, dietician, podiatrist, ophthalmologist).
- Provide emotional support.
- Teach self-monitoring of blood glucose (SMBG).
- Teach S&S of alterations in blood glucose.
- Teach administration of medications (insulin injection, insulin pump).
- Explain need for medical alert ID.

Hypothyroidism

- *Primary hypothyroidism:* Autoimmune lymphocytic destruction (**Hashimoto thyroiditis**), atrophy with aging, genetics, medications (iodides, lithium), toxic effect of hyperthyroidism therapy (thyroidectomy, ^{131}I).
- *Secondary hypothyroidism:* Hypothalamus and/or pituitary problems, causing ↓ thyrotropin-releasing hormone (TRH) or ↓ thyroid-stimulating hormone (TSH).

Signs and Symptoms

- ↓ VS; ↑ weight; dry, pale skin; brittle hair/nails; cold intolerance.
- Constipation, periorbital edema, anemia, enlarged tongue.
- Dull expression, apathy, lethargy.
- ↓ T_3, ↓ T_4, ↑ TSH, ↑ cholesterol, ↓ HDL, ↑ LDL.
- Severe hypothyroidism (**myxedema**) may cause coma.

Treatment

- Hormone replacement with levothyroxine.
- TSH levels are monitored as dose is gradually ↑ to determine optimum dose.

Nursing Care

- Assess for S&S; explain that symptoms will improve with hormonal replacement.
- Teach to ↑ rest, measures to stay warm; ↑ fluids and fiber to ↓ constipation.
- Teach S&S of hyperthyroidism that may result from excessive hormonal replacement.
- Assess for toxic effects of medications especially CNS depressants due to ↓ metabolism.

Hyperthyroidism (Graves Disease, Thyrotoxicosis)

- Excessive production of thyroid hormones; T_3 (triiodothyronine) and T_4 (thyroxine); caused by stimulation of thyroid gland by circulating immunoglobulins; has an autoimmune component; often precipitated by stress or infection, resulting in ↑ metabolic rate and sensitivity to catecholamines.
- Generally occurs between 20–40 yr of age; more common in females.
- Sudden, severe, life-threatening hyperthyroidism known as **thyroid storm** or **thyrotoxic crisis**.
- Can precipitate osteoporosis, amenorrhea, heart failure.

Signs and Symptoms

- ↑VS, ↑ BP, hunger, ↓ weight, diarrhea, enlargement of gland **(goiter)**.
- Tremors, nervousness, bulging eyes **(exophthalmos)**.
- ↑ sweating, flushed skin, heat intolerance.
- Increase in radioactive iodine uptake, T_3, and T_4; ↓TSH.
- *Thyroid storm/thyrotoxic crisis:* ↑T, P >120 bpm, delirium, heart failure, coma.

Treatment

- Radioactive iodine (^{131} I) destroys thyroid cells.
- Propylthiouracil (PRU) or methimazole (Tapazol) to ↓T_4.
- Subtotal thyroidectomy; proceeded by iodine therapy (potassium iodide, SSKI) to ↓ vascularity.

Nursing Care

- Assess for S&S of thyroid storm/thyrotoxic crisis.
- Provide calm, cool environment; high-protein, high-calorie diet.
- Teach S&S of hypothyroidism that may result from treatment.
- Administer eye care (drops, taping eyes shut when sleeping) for exophthalmos.
- *Thyroid storm/thyrotoxic crisis:* Maintain hypothermia blanket; administer prescribed oxygen (O_2), propranolol, steroids, propylthiouracil and/or iodide.

Cardiovascular Disorders

Ischemic Heart Disease (IHD): Angina and Myocardial Infarction

Angina
- Fatty deposits in intima of coronary arteries precipitate inflammatory process → plaques **(atheromas)** → further obstruction of blood flow → chest pain due to myocardial ischemia.

Myocardial Infarction (MI)
- Rupture of atheroma → thrombus → severe ischemia and myocardial cell death.
- Other causes of MIs include ↓ myocardial oxygen supply (vasospasm, hemorrhage), ↑ oxygen demand (cocaine, hyperthyroidism).

Risk Factors
- Aging, family history, race (African ancestry), gender (males more than premenopausal females).
- Hypertension (HTN), DM, metabolic syndrome (insulin resistance, abdominal obesity, abnormal lipid profile).
- Modifiable risk factors: Smoking, obesity, sedentary lifestyle.
- ↑ cholesterol, ↑ triglycerides, ↑ LDL, ↓ HDL, ↑ C-reactive protein (CRP).

Signs and Symptoms
Angina
- Chest pain/pressure may be substernal and/or radiate to neck, jaw, left arm.
- Precipitated by exertion (↑ oxygen demand); cold exposure (vasoconstriction); stress (sympathetic nervous system [SNS] activity → ↑ oxygen demand); heavy meal (blood diverted to GI tract decreases blood to heart).
- Pain subsides with rest and/or nitroglycerin.

Myocardial Infarction
- May have sudden chest pain (see Angina) unrelieved by rest/nitroglycerin.
- SOB; restlessness; cool, pale, clammy skin; diaphoresis; N&V.
- Pulse deficit if atrial fibrillation.
- *Early S&S in women:* Overwhelming fatigue, dizziness, indigestion, anxiety, insomnia.

Diagnostic Tests
- ECG: ↑ ST segment, inverted T wave, presence of Q wave.
- Echocardiogram: Identifies ↓ ventricular wall motion and ↓ ejection fraction.
- Myoglobin: ↑ in 1–3 hr, returns to baseline in 12 hr.

- Isoenzyme specific to heart muscle damage:
  - Cardiac troponin T (cTnT): ↑ in 3–6 hr and remains ↑ 14–21 days.
  - Cardiac troponin I (cTnI): ↑ in 7–14 hr and remains ↑ 5–7 days.
  - CK–MB: ↑ in 4–6 hr, returns to baseline in 3 days.

Treatment
- ↓ cardiac demands and ↑ oxygen to cardiac muscle.

Angina
- ↓ modifiable risk factors; percutaneous coronary interventional (PCI) procedures (PCTA, atherectomy, stent); coronary artery bypass graft (CABG).
- Meds: Nitroglycerin, beta-blockers, calcium channel blockers, antiplatelets, anticoagulants, antilipidemics.
- Oxygen prn; cardiac rehab to ↑ exercise tolerance and quality of life.

Myocardial Infarction
- Provide oxygen; morphine to ↓ pain.
- IV thrombolytics within 3 hr of start of MI to dissolve clot and ↓ damage.
- Meds: Opioid analgesics, beta-blockers, ACE inhibitors, stool softeners, anticoagulants.
- Emergency PCI; additional care (see Angina above).

Nursing Care
Angina
- Assess for S&S; balance activity/rest; give sublingual nitroglycerin and oxygen prn.
- Teach medications; teach to ↓ modifiable risk factors.

Myocardial Infarction
- Assess cardiac function (ECG, hemodynamic parameters, arterial blood gases); ↑ head of bed (HOB); administer prescribed oxygen and opioid.
- Maintain IV access; avoid fluid overload; maintain bedrest (BR) until stable.
- Identify S&S of complications: Heart failure, pulmonary edema, dysrhythmias, cardiogenic shock.
- **Percutaneous transluminal coronary angioplasty (PCTA)**
  - Assess for bleeding (restlessness, back pain due to retroperitoneal bleed, ↑ P, ↓ BP, ↓ Hb, ↓ Hct).
  - Apply pressure to insertion site; keep limb extended.
- Assess distal pulses of extremity.
- **Postoperative coronary artery bypass graft (CABG)**
  - Assess hemodynamic status, which may be ↑ due to heart failure or fluid overload or ↓ due to fluid deficit or bleeding.
  - Assess pulses distal to vein harvest site if a lower extremity vein is used.
  - Monitor ECG for dysrhythmias.
  - Assess urine output; notify primary health-care provider if <30 mL/hr because it may indicate ↓ renal perfusion.

- Monitor electrolytes and coagulation profile.
- Maintain chest tube drainage and ventilator as needed, then encourage incentive spirometer, splinting, coughing, and deep breathing.
- Provide for alternate communication while intubated.
- Provide pain control.
- Refer to cardiac rehab and Mended Hearts Club.

Hypertension (HTN)

- Increased systolic blood pressure (SBP) and/or increased diastolic blood pressure (DBP).
- *Prehypertension:* SBP 120–139 mm Hg, DBP 80–89 mm Hg.
- *Stage 1:* SBP 140–159 mm Hg, DBP 90–99 mm Hg.
- *Stage 2:* SBP ≥160 mm Hg, DBP ≥100 mm Hg.
- ↑ peripheral resistance; ↑ cardiac output, and/or ↑ blood volume due to ↑ renin, ↑ angiotensin, ↑ aldosterone, Na, and water retention, ↑ SNS activity, pregnancy, medications, renal disease.
- HTN → vascular changes → ventricular hypertrophy, heart failure, MI, kidney disease, retinopathy.
- *Preload:* Stretch of cardiac muscle fibers at end of diastole.
- *Afterload:* Resistance to ejection of blood from left ventricle.

Treatment
- Lifestyle modifications (see Nursing Care below).
- Medications such as diuretics, beta-blockers, alpha-blockers, ACE inhibitors, angiotensin II receptor blockers, calcium channel blockers, vasodilators, antilipidemics.

Nursing Care
- Assess BP and S&S of target organ damage (SOB, angina, ↓ vision, epistaxis, headache, edema).
- Teach health promotion: ↓ smoking, ↓ weight, ↓ alcohol intake, ↑ aerobic activity, ↓ stress.
- Teach balanced diet with restrictions in Na, saturated fats, cholesterol; ↑ fruits, vegetables, whole grains, fish, poultry, nuts in diet.

Heart Failure (HF)

- Cardiac output insufficient due to ↓ ventricular filling (diastolic HF) or ↓ ventricular contraction (systolic HF).
- Decreased cardiac output stimulates SNS → ↑ cardiac workload and ventricular hypertrophy → ↓ renal perfusion.
- ↓ renal perfusion → renin/angiotensin response → vasoconstriction and ↑ aldosterone.

- ↑ aldosterone → Na and water retention → further ↑ cardiac workload.
- Pressure may ↑ in pulmonary circulation (**left**-sided HF) or in systemic circulation (**right-sided HF**).
- Severe HF may → cardiomegaly, pulmonary edema, and/or cardiogenic shock.

Risk Factors
- Coronary artery disease; inflammation/infection of cardiac structures.
- Structural disorders of valves (mitral regurgitation, aortic stenosis).
- Dysrhythmias such as rapid atrial fibrillation.
- ↑ cardiac demands related to HTN, anemia, thyrotoxicosis, fever, obesity, excessive alcohol intake.

Signs and Symptoms
- ↑ P, ↑ R, fatigue, dyspnea, restlessness, confusion, third heart sound (**ventricular gallop**), cardiomegaly, ↓ urine output.
- *S&S of systemic circulation congestion:* Ankle edema, anorexia, nausea, hepatomegaly, ascites, jugular vein distention.
- *S&S of pulmonic circulation congestion:* Crackles, cyanosis, frothy sputum.

Diagnostic Tests
- ↑ brain natriuretic peptide (BNP); ↑ *N*-terminal prohormone (NT-proBNP); these neurohormones are released in response to hemodynamic stress.
- Echocardiogram, chest x-ray to identify cardiomegaly.

Treatment
- Treat cause (PTCA for ischemic heart disease [IHD]), oxygen, ventricular pacing.
- ACE inhibitors to ↓ preload and ↓ afterload.
- Beta-blockers to counteract SNS overstimulation.
- Diuretics to ↓ fluid overload, digoxin to ↑ cardiac output.
- *Acute heart failure:* Intubation, mechanical ventilation, and positive end-expiratory pressure (PEEP) to ↓ hypoxia; diuretics; opioid; cardiac stimulant to ↑ cardiac output.

Nursing Care
- Assess apical pulse for galloping rhythm; radial pulse for rate, rhythm, volume; compare apical and radial pulses for pulse deficit; daily weight; breath sounds (crackles).
- Teach to ↓ smoking, ↓ weight, gradually ↑ exercise, ↓ Na in diet, ↑ potassium in diet (dried fruit, bananas, oranges, melon).
- ↑ HOB to ↓ venous return; give oxygen; teach about medications.

Anemia

- ■ Features common to all types of anemia (see Tab 4, PEDS, Anemia, p. 123, for iron deficiency, sickle cell, and β-thalassemia).
- ■ ↓ RBCs due to blood loss, ↓ production or ↑ destruction of RBCs, ↓ oxygen carrying capacity of blood, ↑ cardiac workload, heart failure.
- ■ *S&S:* ↑ P, ↑ R, fatigue, weakness, pallor, confusion, ↓ Hb, ↓ Hct.

Treatment
Correct cause; provide oxygen; administer transfusions (whole blood, packed RBCs) and medications depending on type of anemia.

Nursing Care
Asses for S&S; balance rest/activity; ↑ protein, fiber and fluids in diet; teach iron supplements will cause black stools and constipation; administer ordered blood products.

Microcytic Anemia
- ■ ↓ iron due to ↓ dietary intake (vegetarians, teens); blood loss from GI bleeding (ulcers, cancer, inflammation) or menorrhagia; ↓ iron absorption after gastric surgery.
- ■ *S&S:* Mean corpuscular volume (MCV) <80 fL; ↓ ferritin; ↓ serum iron; ↓ transferrin; inflammation of tongue **(glossitis)** and lip **(cheilitis)**; craving for ice, clay, starch, etc. **(pica)**.

Treatment and Nursing Care
Give oral iron with orange juice between meals (vitamin C and empty stomach ↑ absorption); dilute liquid iron, use straw, and rinse mouth after administration (stains teeth); ↑ dietary sources of iron, such as raisins, eggs, meat (liver), green vegetables.

Macrocytic Anemia
- ■ ↓ folate due to ↓ dietary intake, alcohol; B_{12} deficiency due to lack of intrinsic factor **(pernicious anemia)**; ↓ folate absorption after gastric surgery or Crohn disease.
- ■ *S&S:* MCV >100 fL; ↓ folate; ↓ B_{12} (Schilling test for pernicious anemia); sore, smooth, red, tongue; diarrhea; neurological changes due to ↓ myelin (paresthesias, ataxia); screen for stomach Ca.

Treatment and Nursing Care
Give oral folic acid; intramuscular (IM) B_{12}; teach to avoid alcohol; ↑ dietary sources of folic acid (green vegetables, liver, mushrooms).

Normocytic Anemia
- *Hemolytic anemia (HA):* RBCs break down rapidly → ↑ bone marrow release of reticulocytes; examples include G-6-PD deficiency, toxins that precipitate HA, sickle cell anemia, β-thalassemia.
- *Anemia in renal disease:* ↓ erythropoietin → ↓ RBCs synthesis.
- *S&S:* MCV 80–100 fL; ↑ reticulocytes; jaundice due to Hb breakdown; hepatomegaly; S&S of acute hemolysis (↑T, chills, abdominal and back pain, hemoglobinuria).

Treatment and Nursing Care
- *HA:* Depends on etiology.
- *Renal disease:* Iron, folate, recombinant erythropoietin.

Arterial Insufficiency

Atherosclerosis → ischemia of extremities (↑ incidence in distal legs); ↓ sensation → ↑ risk of injury.

Risk Factors
- ↑ age, males, heredity, smoking, obesity, inactivity, HTN, hyperlipidemia, diabetes.

Signs and Symptoms
- Leg pain when walking relieved by rest **(intermittent claudication)**.
- Cool, pale, shiny leg with faint/absent pulse.
- ↓ hair on legs; thick, yellow toenails; ulcers on toes that may extend to dry gangrene.

Treatment
- ↓ risk factors.
- Anticoagulants to ↓ platelet aggregation and bypass grafts to ↑ blood flow.

Nursing Care
- Assess for S&S.
- Position legs ↓ than heart; keep legs/feet warm (socks, blankets).
- Teach to ↓ smoking and exposure to cold; avoid constrictive clothing.
- Foot care: Inspect feet daily; wear shoes and socks and dry feet well to protect feet; apply ordered dressings to ulcers.

Aortic Aneurysm

Weakness in vessel → protrusion and possible rupture.

Risk Factors
- Atherosclerosis, trauma, congenital weakness, infection, inflammation, HTN, smoking.

Signs and Symptoms
- May be symptom-free; may be able to palpate a pulsating mass.
- Diagnosis confirmed with CT, MRI, sonogram.
- *Dissecting aneurysm:* Sudden severe chest pain extending to back, shoulder, epigastrium, abdomen; diaphoresis; ↑ P.

Treatment
- Surgical repair with graft.
- Antihypertensives to ↓ BP and risk of extension or rupture.

Nursing Care
- Assess BP; monitor Hb and Hct.
- Assess for sudden ↑ pain that may signal impending rupture.
- Teach to avoid activities that ↑ intra-abdominal pressure (sneezing, coughing, vomiting, straining at stool).

Deep Vein Thrombosis (DVT)

Virchow triad: Venous stasis, damage to vein, ↑ blood coagulation.

Risk Factors
- ↑ age, obesity, immobility, oral contraceptives, varicose veins, popliteal pressure, fractures.

Signs and Symptoms
- Edema, ache, calf pain on foot dorsiflexion **(Homan sign)**; Homan sign should not be elicited deliberately because it may cause a thrombus to become an embolus.
- ↑ P, dyspnea, chest pain if thrombus dislodges, causing a pulmonary embolus (PE).

Treatment
- Thrombolytics, anticoagulants.
- Thrombectomy; insertion of vena cava filter to prevent PE.

Nursing Care
- *Prevention:* Provide antiembolism stockings, sequential compression device, encourage exercise, ↑ fluids, give prophylactic anticoagulant.
- *Acute phase:* Maintain bedrest, elevate extremity, apply ordered warm soaks, give prescribed anticoagulant.

Venous Insufficiency

Incompetent valves and ↑ venous pressure → vein dilation; ↓ sensation → ↑ risk of injury.

Risk Factors
- Varicose veins, thrombophlebitis, aging, inactivity (lack of muscle contraction).

Signs and Symptoms
- Leg edema, pain, fatigue, and heaviness that ↑ over day.
- Brownish pigmentation of legs **(hemosiderin deposition)**.
- Stasis ulcers with exudate around ankles and lower legs.

Treatment
- Positioning, compression therapy (Unna boot, Velcro wrap) to ↓ venous pressure; antibiotics if infection occurs.
- Surgical and nonsurgical débridement of necrotic tissue.

Nursing Care
- Elevate legs; apply elastic stockings before legs are dependent; teach to avoid constrictive clothing; administer prescribed antibiotics and wound care.
- Foot care: Teach to inspect feet daily, wear shoes and socks, dry feet well (particularly between toes), implement ordered dressings to ulcers.

Respiratory Disorders

Features common to most respiratory disorders:

- ↓ ventilation due to obstruction or ↓ surface area for gas exchange.
- Results in ↓ O_2 to below physiological level **(hypoxia)** and ↑ CO_2 to an excessive level **(hypercapnia)** → ↑ $Paco_2$, ↓ arterial pH **(respiratory acidosis)**.

Signs and Symptoms
- ↑ P, ↑ R, fatigue, weakness, restlessness, confusion.
- Adventitious breath sounds, dyspnea, orthopnea, use of accessory muscles of respiration, ↓ pulse oximetry.

Treatment
Based on cause; oxygen; prophylactic influenza/pneumonia vaccines for those at ↑ risk.

Nursing Care

- Assess for S&S; ↑ HOB, administer oxygen, prescribed medications.
- Teach to balance activity/rest; stop smoking.

Pneumonia

- Microorganisms from upper airway/blood, aspiration of food/gastric contents → inflammation.
- Alveoli fill with exudate and WBCs (**consolidation**) → ↓ ventilation and ↓ diffusion of gases; aerosolized or droplet transmission.

Risk Factors

- ↑↓ age, smoking, immunosuppression.
- Winter (Streptococcal pneumonia); summer and fall (*Legionella*).

Signs and Symptoms

- ↑T and WBCs, adventitious breath sounds, cough, sputum (character depends on organism).
- Chest x-ray indicates patchy or lobe consolidation or infiltrates.

Treatment

- Antibiotic regime based on C&S results that identify organism.
- Replace fluid losses due to ↑T and ↑R.

Nursing Care

- Assess for signs of respiratory distress: ↑R, use of accessory muscles of respiration, dyspnea, ↓LOC.
- Administer ordered chest PT, ↑fluids, oxygen.
- Teach how to prevent recurrence and ↓transmission (hand hygiene, correct tissue disposal).
- Teach need to finish antibiotic regime to ↓recurrence and/or resistance.

Tuberculosis (TB)

- Infection of lungs caused by *Mycobacterium tuberculosis*; granulomas of bacilli become fibrous tissue mass (**Ghon tubercle**) that can calcify and become dormant or ulcerate and activate the bacilli; transmitted via inhalation of infected respiratory droplets.
- *Miliary TB:* Bacilli may travel to bone, kidneys, or brain.

Risk Factors

- ↓immune response (HIV, steroids), crowded living conditions (prisons, long-term care facilities), alcoholism, malnutrition, debilitating physical conditions.

Signs and Symptoms
- Night sweats, ↓ weight, cough, hemoptysis.
- Positive PPD/Mantoux: 10 mm induration indicates immune response (exposure to but not necessarily the disease).
- Chest x-ray reveals active/calcified lesions; acid fast bacteria in sputum.

Treatment
- Combination of antituberculars for 6–12 months (Tab 7, MEDS, Antituberculars, p. 256).
- Prophylactic INH for exposure.

Nursing Care
- Use airborne precautions during active disease.
- Teach need for long-term adherence to medication regimen.
- Teach prevention of transmission to family members: Frequent hand hygiene, use of disposable tissues, covering cough, use of separate eating utensils.

Emphysema

- Alveolar wall becomes distended, inelastic, or destroyed → ↓ effective surface area for gas exchange, air trapping, ↑ residual volume.
- Results in ↑ work to exhale; chronic hypercapnia (↑ $Paco_2$); may cause right-sided heart failure (**cor pulmonale**).

Risk Factors
- ↑ age, smoking, secondhand smoke, inhaled pollutants, alpha-antitrypsin deficiency.

Signs and Symptoms
- Barrel chest, clubbing of fingers, cyanosis, pursed-lip breathing, use of accessory muscles of respiration.
- ↓ forced expiratory volume, ↑ residual volume.

Treatment
- Smoking cessation.
- O_2 at less than 2 L/min because with emphysema excessive exogenous O_2 ↓ the respiratory drive and results in ↓ breathing and ↑ CO_2 retention. Normally ↑ CO_2 stimulates breathing. With emphysema, there is chronic ↑ CO_2 and as a result, low O_2 stimulates breathing. In addition, the Haldane effect suggests that the adverse effects of ↑ O_2 are caused by the inability of oxygen-saturated hemoglobin molecules to transport CO_2. Both issues relate to CO_2 narcosis.
- Steroids, bronchodilators, lung volume reduction, lung transplant.

Nursing Care

- Maintain oxygen at ≤2 L.
- Teach diaphragmatic and pursed-lip breathing to extend exhalation and keep alveoli open.
- Balance activity and rest.

Lung Cancer

- Altered DNA → altered cellular replication; may be primary or metastatic; often metastasizes to lymph nodes, bone, brain before diagnosis.
- Types: Adenocarcinoma, small cell (oat cell), large cell (undifferentiated), squamous cell carcinoma.

Risk Factors

- Inhalation of carcinogens (tobacco smoke, asbestos, exposure to radon).
- Heredity, primary cancer at another site.

Signs and Symptoms

- Dry, chronic cough; hoarseness; ↓ weight; lymphadenopathy.
- Sputum positive for cytology.
- Chest x-ray indicates lesion and possible effusion.
- Biopsy indicates source (primary or secondary).

Treatment

- Thoracentesis with chest x-ray before/after, lobectomy, pneumonectomy.
- Chemotherapy, radiation, palliative care to ↓ pain.

Nursing Care

- Lobectomy: Manage chest tubes.
- Pneumonectomy: Place on operative side.
- Chemotherapy: Manage side effects (see Nursing Care for Patients With Cancer or Experiencing Nontherapeutic Effects of Antineoplastic Therapies, p. 178).
- Thoracentesis: Assess respiratory status before/after (pneumothorax and subcutaneous emphysema are complications); support patient in orthopneic position during procedure; tell patient to hold breath during needle insertion; position on opposite side of insertion for 1 hr after.
- Support decision for hospice or palliative care.

Acute Respiratory Distress Syndrome (ARDS)

- Direct or indirect lung trauma → inflammation → fluid movement into alveolar spaces and ↓ surfactant → atelectasis → hypoxia and ↑ dead space.
- Due to trauma, aspiration, shock, infection.

Signs and Symptoms

- Early: Dyspnea, anxiety, $\downarrow O_2$ sat, $\downarrow Pao_2$.
- Late: $\uparrow CO_2$, cyanosis, lung infiltrate on x-ray.

Treatment

- Treat cause; mechanical ventilation and PEEP keeps alveoli open.
- Steroids, interleukin-1 receptor antagonists, surfactant therapy.
- Sedatives or neuromuscular blocks to $\downarrow$ fighting the ventilator.

Nursing Care

- Assess for S&S, arterial blood gases, oxygen saturation; suction airway.
- Patient on a mechanical ventilator:
  - Assess breath sounds: Absence indicates pneumothorax due to PEEP; unilateral aeration indicates endotracheal tube (ET) may be in one bronchi (usually right).
  - Maintain trach or ET cuff pressure seal to ensure full volume delivery.
  - Check ventilator settings and alarms; high-pressure alarm responds to obstruction due to mucus or tubing kinks; low-pressure alarm responds to $\downarrow$ cuff pressure or separation of tubing.
  - Provide alternate mode of communication.

Pneumothorax

- Disruption of lining of lung (**visceral pleura**) or lining of thoracic cavity (**parietal pleura**) permitting air (**pneumothorax**) and/or blood (**hemothorax**) into pleural space → lung collapse.
- Due to rib fracture, stab or gunshot wound, thoracentesis, emphysema.

Signs and Symptoms

- Sudden unilateral chest pain; air/blood in pleural space on x-ray.
- $\uparrow P$, $\uparrow R$, dyspnea, $\downarrow$ breath sounds on affected side, $\downarrow Pao_2$.

Treatment

- Oxygen, insertion of chest tube/water seal drainage to reestablish negative pressure (pneumothorax—2nd anterior intercostal space, hemothorax—lower and more posterior space).

Nursing Care

- Assess for S&S; relieve pain.
- Assess water seal chamber fluid level ($\uparrow$ on inspiration and $\downarrow$ with exhalation) and for bubbling in water seal chamber (continuous bubbling suggests air leak and absence suggests full lung expansion or blocked tube).
- Instruct patient to exhale and bear down when removing chest tube, then apply occlusive dressing.
- *Subcutaneous emphysema:* Palpate around insertion site for crackles, which indicates air in subcutaneous tissue (**crepitus**).

Asthma

See Tab 4, PEDS, Asthma, p. 117

Musculoskeletal Disorders

Fractures

- Break in bone continuity from excessive force. Traumatizes muscles, blood vessels, and nerves leading to inflammation and possible hemorrhage.
- Types of fractures:
  - *Simple (closed):* Skin remains intact.
  - *Compound (open):* Fragments penetrate skin.
  - *Transverse:* Straight across.
  - *Oblique:* Angled across.
  - *Spiral:* Twists around shaft.
  - *Comminuted:* Multiple bone fragments.
  - *Compression:* Compressed bone mass.
  - *Depressed:* Bone fragments forced inward.
  - *Greenstick:* Break partially extends across and then along length; common in children.
  - *Pathological:* Less force than usual needed to break bone due to ↑ age; porous, brittle bones (**osteoporosis**); metastatic or primary tumors; Paget disease.

Signs and Symptoms

- Pain, spasms, shortening of extremity, ecchymosis.
- Grating sound when moved (**crepitus**).
- ↓ mobility, deformity, paresthesias due to nerve damage.
- Shock due to hemorrhage.
- *Fat emboli:* Dyspnea; ↑ VS; copious white sputum; crackles; ↓ mentation; buccal, conjunctival, and chest petechiae.
- *Compartment syndrome:* ↑ muscle compartment pressure due to edema/bleeding → ↓ circulation → tissue hypoxia → ↑ pain and damage.

Treatment

- Closed reduction: Bone fragments aligned and stabilized with cast, splint, traction.
- Open reduction internal fixation (ORIF): Bone fragments stabilized with wires, pins, nails, rods, plates.
- Total hip replacement: Surgical insertion of a prosthetic system with hardware for each surface of the joint.

Nursing Care

- Immobilize to ↓ trauma and pain; pain management.
- *Peripheral neurovascular assessment of extremity:* ↓ peripheral pulses; pallor; cool to touch; capillary refill >2–3 sec; ↓ motor/sensory function; may extend to ↓ muscle perfusion due to ↑ tissue pressure within closed fascial compartment **(compartment syndrome)**; elevate limb and notify health-care provider of impaired status.
- *Patient with a cast:* ↑ on pillow; uncover to ↑ drying; handle with palms not fingertips until dry; encourage isometric exercise to ↓ atrophy; odor may indicate infection.
- *Patient with traction:* Hang weights freely; maintain functional alignment; provide ordered pin care for skeletal traction.
- *Patient with external fixation device:* Observe for S&S of infection at pin sites; provide ordered pin care; support limb when moving patient; encourage use of nonrestrictive clothing.
- *Postoperative care for patient after total hip replacement:*
  - Manage pain: patient-controlled analgesia; IM, sub-Q, oral opioids.
  - Avoid displacement of prosthesis: Abduction pillow and high toilet seat/chair; avoid internal rotation or hip flexion >90°.
  - Prevent DVT: Anticoagulants, compression devices, avoidance of dorsiflexion, popliteal pressure.
  - Prevent atelectasis/pneumonia: Incentive spirometry; coughing and deep breathing.

Rheumatoid Arthritis (RA)	Osteoarthritis (OA)	Gouty Arthritis
• Immune response → inflammation, breakdown of collagen, synovial edema, pannus formation, narrowed joint space, bone spurs.	• Involves chondrocyte response → cartilage breakdown.	• Purine metabolism defect → ↑ serum uric acid → urate deposits that become porous stone **(tophi)**.
Risk Factors		
• ↑ in female.	• ↑ age, obesity, joint injury, repetitive use, congenital hip subluxation.	• Starvation, organ meat and shell-fish intake, ↑ cell proliferation (leukemia, psoriasis), ↑ in males.
Signs and Symptoms		
• Acute bilateral inflammation of joints (hands, wrists, feet, and later other joints). • Pain unrelieved by rest; a.m. stiffness longer than 1 hr. • Deformities (ulnar drift, swan neck, Boutonniere deformity). • ↑ erythrocyte sedimentation rate (ESR), ↑ C-reactive protein, ↑ rheumatoid factor, ↑ antinuclear antibody (ANA); synovial fluid has complements and WBCs. • Fatigue, anemia, ↑T, ↑ node size.	• Morning stiffness of hips, knees, cervica /lumbar spine, small joints of hands and feet for less than1 hr; improves with activity. • Bony hypertrophy occurring in fingers **(Heberden, Bouchard nodes)**; if inflamed, they enlarge and are tender, joint spaces narrow, crepitus occurs with joint movement.	• Acute asymmetric joint pain and inflammation. • Located most often in big toe but may affect ankle, knee, elbow, wrist, or fingers. • Tophi in periphery (outer ear, feet, hands, elbows, knees). • ↑ serum uric acid, uric acid crystals in synovial fluid, urate renal calculi and nephropathy.

Treatment		
Rheumatoid Arthritis (RA)	**Osteoarthritis (OA)**	**Gouty Arthritis**
• Meds: Steroids, NSAIDs, disease-modifying antirheumatic drugs (DMARDs). • Synovectomy; joint fusion or replacement.	• Meds: Acetaminophen, glucosamine and chondroitin, topical capsaicin; knee-joint injections of hyaluronic acid. • Arthroplasty.	• Meds: Colchicine (Colsalide), probenecid (Benemid), allopurinol (Zyloprim). • ↓ intake of purines (organ meats) and alcohol. • ↑ fluid intake to ↓ renal calculi.

Nursing Care: Balance rest/activity; provide or teach ROM; keep joints in functional alignment; apply ordered heat or cold; give prescribed meds; implement nondrug pain relief measures; encourage ↓ weight; teach use of adaptive devices to ↑ independence; refer to Arthritis Foundation.

Neurological Disorders

Multiple Sclerosis

■ Autoimmune response → formation of scattered sclerotic plaques on demyelinated axons → ↓ impulse conduction.
■ Remissions and exacerbations with downward plateaus.
■ Frequently affected areas: Optic nerves, cerebrum, brain stem, cerebellum, spinal cord.

Risk Factors
■ Caucasian race 20–40 yr of age; female gender.

Signs and Symptoms
■ Vary depending on nerves involved.
■ Charcot triad: Intention tremor, nystagmus, scanning speech.
■ Visual disturbances: Diplopia, visual field deficits.
■ Fatigue, paresthesias, dysphagia, incoordination, slurred speech, spasticity, bladder dysfunction, emotional lability.

Treatment
■ Disease-modifying therapy (interferon beta-1a and -1b, glatiramer acetate).
■ Corticosteroids, antispasmodics.
■ Palliative care: PT, OT.

Nursing Care
■ Assess for S&S, balance activity/rest, provide cool environment.
■ Ensure safe mobility: Wide base of support, assistive devices.
■ Prevent pressure ulcers: Change position every 1–2 hr, skin care, pull sheet to ↓ shearing, pressure-relieving devices.
■ Improve elimination pattern: Respond to urge, follow bowel and bladder toileting schedule, ↑ fiber and fluids, give prescribed ascorbic acid to acidify urine.
■ Encourage PT, ↓ fat in diet.
■ Encourage ventilation of feelings, refer to National Multiple Sclerosis Society.

Seizures

■ Sudden, abnormal electrical discharge from cerebral neurons → generalized seizures (affect both hemispheres) or partial seizure (start in one area of the brain).
■ Secondary to cerebrovascular disease, head trauma, brain tumor, drug or alcohol withdrawal, hypoglycemia, high temperature in children.

Signs and Symptoms

Partial (Focal, Local) Seizures
- *Simple:* Single muscle movement (twitch) or sensory alteration, remains conscious, may report an aura.
- *Complex:* Sensory, motor, or autonomic response with altered LOC for 1–3 min; associated with blank stare; lack of attention to verbal stimuli; and chewing, swallowing, fumbling movements; no memory of event following seizure.

Generalized Seizures
- **Tonic-clonic (formerly grand mal seizure)**
- Intense muscle contractions (tonic phase); alternating with relaxation (clonic phase).
- Often proceeded by flash of light or specific noise (**aura**).
- Unconsciousness, shallow/absent breathing, bladder/bowel incontinence.
- Confusion, drowsiness, and/or sleep following seizure.
- **Absence (formerly petit mal seizure)**
  - Abrupt, brief (3–5 sec) loss of consciousness.
  - More common in children; may disappear at puberty.
- **Myoclonic**
  - Short (few min) sporadic periods of muscle contractions.
  - Often secondary seizures; rare.
- **Tonic**
  - Increase in muscle tone; loss of consciousness.
  - Autonomic changes for 30 sec to several minutes.
- **Atonic**
  - Sudden loss of muscle tone for several seconds; confusion after event.
- **Clonic**
  - Muscle contraction and relaxation lasting several minutes.
- **Status epilepticus**
  - Continuous tonic-clonic seizure activity for >30 min; life-threatening.
- **Febrile**
  - Tonic-clonic seizure with T >101.8°F; most common in children; self-limiting.

Treatment
- Antiseizure agents, treatment of underlying cause (e.g., brain tumor, fever).

Nursing Care
- Assess seizure activity: Precipitating event, presence of aura, specific origin and progression of motor activity, length, patient response.
- Identify presence of status epilepticus.
- Protect patient: Ease to floor if out of bed, protect head, loosen clothes, do not insert airway or restrain patient, position laterally if possible.
- Teach need to adhere to antiseizure therapy to maintain therapeutic levels; continue health-care supervision; wear medical alert band.

- Teach to avoid factors that may precipitate a seizure (flickering lights, alcohol, sleep deprivation, excessive exercise, emotional stress).
- Provide emotional support related to patient's concerns (fear of seizure, stigmatization, incontinence during a seizure, inability to drive until condition is controlled); refer to Epilepsy Foundation of America.

Parkinson Disease

- Neuronal destruction of substantia nigra in basal ganglia → ↓ dopamine → neurotransmitter imbalance.
- Progressive degeneration; may lead to complete dependence.

Risk Factors
- Genetics, male gender, 50–60 yr of age, atherosclerosis.

Signs and Symptoms
- Pill-rolling motion of thumb against fingers (**resting, nonintention tremor**).
- Propulsive, shuffling gait (**cogwheel gait**); no arm swing; slow voluntary movement (**bradykinesia**).
- Stooped posture, masklike facies, rigidity, monotone voice, dysphagia, constipation, incontinence, ↑ cognition.

Treatment
- *Anti-Parkinson agents:* Dopaminergics, anticholinergics, antivirals, dopamine agonist, MAO inhibitors.
- Deep brain stimulation, destruction of thalamus for tremor and globus pallidus for bradykinesia.
- Palliative care: PT, OT.

Nursing Care
- Maintain airway, suction as needed.
- Provide safe mobility: Wide base of support, assistive devices, encourage to walk erect and take longer steps, balance activity and rest.
- Provide warm baths and active ROM to ↑ rigidity; splints to ↓ contractures.
- Promote bowel elimination: ↑ fluids, ↑ roughage, raised toilet seat.
- Promote nutrition: Assistive devices, bite-size pieces, thicken liquids.
- Provide emotional support: ↑ ventilation of feelings; refer to National Parkinson Foundation.

Myasthenia Gravis	Guillain-Barré Syndrome	Amyotrophic Lateral Sclerosis (ALS; Lou Gehrig Disease)
• Autoimmune response → antibody attachment to acetylcholine receptor sites causing destruction of acetylcholine → ↓ impulse transmission → muscle weakness that worsens with activity and improves with rest; remissions and exacerbations.	• Autoimmune response → ascending peripheral nerve myelin destruction → ↓ ability to transmit impulses. • Schwann cells eventually produce myelin → recovery, but may take 2 yr and leave residual deficits.	• Cause unknown; possible autoimmune response or excess nerve stimulation by glutamate → progressive loss of upper and lower motor neurons → lack of muscle stimulation → progressive muscle atrophy. • Life expectancy about 3–5 yr.
Risk Factors		
• Females, 20–40 yr of age; males, 60–70 yr of age.	• Vaccination, recent infection, pregnancy.	• Males, 50–60 yr of age.

Continued

	Myasthenia Gravis	Guillain-Barré Syndrome	Amyotrophic Lateral Sclerosis (ALS; Lou Gehrig Disease)
Signs and Symptoms			
	• Double vision (**diplopia**), eyelid droop (**ptosis**), snarl (**myasthenic smile**), voice change (**dysphonia**). • **Myasthenic crisis:** General weakness, aphagia, respiratory failure.	• Ascending symmetrical weakness/paralysis, areflexia, paresthesias; respiratory paralysis; aphagia; autonomic nerve dysfunction → labile P and BP rates.	• Fatigue, weakness, impaired coordination, muscle twitching (**fasciculations**), nasal-sounding voice, ↑ deep tendon reflexes, dysarthria, dysphagia, dyspnea.
Treatment			
	• Anticholinesterase agents (neostigmine, pyridostigmine), steroids, plasmapheresis, thymectomy to ↓ antibodies.	• IgG IV, oxygen, plasmapheresis, tracheostomy and mechanical ventilation; interventions to prevent complications of immobility such as anticoagulants, compression devices.	• Riluzole, a glutamate antagonist, may prolong life; antispasmodics (baclofen); enteral feedings; mechanical ventilation.

Nursing Care

- Support respirations: Assess respiratory status and oxygen saturation; Fowler position; suctioning; chest PT; incentive spirometer; maintain ET tube, tracheostomy, mechanical ventilator if present.
- Prevent DVT and PE: ROM; prevent popliteal pressure; provide sequential compression devices and anticoagulant as prescribed.
- Prevent pressure ulcers: Reposition every 1–2 hr, skin care, pull sheet to ↓ shearing, pressure-relieving devices.
- Support nutrition: Assess weight; assist with oral intake and prevent aspiration (↑ HOB, feed slowly, use thickening product); provide ordered parenteral or enteral feedings.
- Recognize LOC and mental status are not affected but may be unable to speak.
- Devise alternate means of communication.
- Refer to MG Foundation, GB Foundation, or ALS Association.
- **Myasthenia gravis**
  - Distinguish between myasthenic and cholinergic crises; both cause respiratory muscle weakness, inability to swallow (**aphagia**), and difficulty speaking (**dysarthria**).
  - Give prescribed rapid-acting anticholinesterase (improves symptoms of myasthenic crisis and intensifies symptoms of cholinergic crisis).
  - Give medications at precise times and schedule meals at peak action; provide rest periods.

Brain Attack (BA)/Cerebrovascular Accident (CVA)

- Irreversible neurological deficit caused by cerebral ischemia.
- Caused by embolus, thrombus, hemorrhage (subarachnoid or intracerebral bleeding).

Risk Factors

- Transient ischemic attack (TIA) in which deficits last <24 hr; may precede BA.
- ↑ age, male gender, ↑ BP, DM, cardiac disease, hyperlipidemia.
- African heritage, obesity, smoking, oral contraceptives.

Signs and Symptoms

- Based on location/extent of damage.
- *↑ intracranial pressure (ICP):* Headache, restlessness, ↓ LOC, ↑ systolic BP, widening pulse pressure, ↑T, ↓ P, ↓ R, vomiting, vision problems, unilateral pupil changes, seizures.
- *Posturing:* Arms extended and turned in (**extension, decerebrate**); arms flexed, legs internally rotated (**flexion, decorticate**).

- *Motor:* Unilateral weakness (**hemiparesis**) or unilateral paralysis (**hemiplegia**) on side of body opposite to affected side of brain; difficulty swallowing (**dysphagia**).
- *Bowel/bladder:* Constipation; urinary frequency and urgency; incontinence.
- *Sensory:* Unilateral paresthesia, loss of 1/2 visual field (**hemianopsia**); ↓ proprioception.
- *Communication:* ↓ articulation (**dysarthria**); difficulty communicating thoughts in words (**expressive or Broca aphasia**); difficulty understanding communication (**receptive or Wernicke aphasia**).
- *Cognitive/emotional:* Lability of mood, ↓ memory, ↓ attention span, ↓ judgment.

Treatment

- **Prevention**
  - ↓ weight, ↓ fat in diet, smoking cessation.
  - Antihypertensives for HTN, anticoagulant for atrial fibrillation (AF), glucose control for DM.
  - Carotid endarterectomy.
- **Acute phase**
  - Thrombolytic therapy with tissue plasminogen activator (t-PA) within 3 hr and anticoagulants for ischemic BA.
  - Steroids to ↓ ICP due to cerebral edema.
  - PT, OT, speech therapy, NGT feedings if necessary.
- **Rehabilitation phase:** Multidisciplinary depending on needs.

Nursing Care

- Assess for S&S, balance activity/rest, maintain semi-Fowler position to ↓ ICP.
- Employ seizure precautions: Bed in ↓ position, quiet environment, pad side rails.
- Prevent aspiration: Suction to maintain patent airway; feed slowly; ensure mouth is empty between each mouthful and at end of meal; thicken liquids; ↑ HOB when giving ordered enteral tube feedings.
- Maintain mobility/prevent contractures: ROM, position changes, splints.
- Prevent DVT: Give prescribed anticoagulants, ↓ popliteal pressure, ROM, sequential compression devices, leg exercises.
- Prevent pressure ulcers: Position change every 1–2 hr, skin care, pull sheet to ↓ shearing, pressure relief devices.
- Promote communication: Use picture board, simple sentences with visual clues for receptive aphasia, have patience and avoid completing patient's message for expressive aphasia.
- Support elimination: Respond to urge; bowel and bladder training.
- Involve patient with planning; accept emotional lability and expressions of grieving for losses.

Spinal Cord Injury

- Injury due to contusion, compression, laceration, transection.
- Edema and bleeding → ischemia → ↑ injury.
- Frequently affects C5–7, T12–L1.

Risk Factors

- < 30 yr of age; male gender.
- Automobile collision, violence, falls, diving accident, contact sports, tumors.

Signs and Symptoms

- Varies depending on level of injury.
- *Spinal shock:* Flaccid paralysis; loss of sensation and reflexes below injury; loss of bowel and bladder function.
- *Neurogenic shock:* ↓ BP, ↓ P, inability to sweat due to ↓ autonomic nerve activity.
- *Paralysis:* Depends on level of injury; all four extremities **(quadriplegia)**; both legs **(paraplegia)**.
- *Bladder dysfunction:*
  - *Spastic bladder:* Empties automatically when detrusor muscle is stretched; occurs with injury above conus medullaris.
  - *Flaccid bladder:* Atonic bladder distends and periodically overflows but does not empty; occurs with injury at or below conus medullaris.
- *Autonomic hyperreflexia:*
  - Exaggerated SNS response with cord injury ≥T6.
  - Mainly due to bladder or bowel distention.
  - Headache, ↑ BP, ↓ P, "goose bumps" **(piloerection)**, nasal congestion, diaphoresis, nausea.
- *Respiratory paralysis:* Lack of voluntary breathing with injury above C3–4.

Treatment

- Stabilize head, neck, and spine on backboard for transport.
- IV corticosteroids to ↓ cerebral edema.
- Respiratory support due to paralyzed or weak intercostal muscles.
- Surgery to ↓ compression, correct alignment, ↑ spine stability.
- Traction with skeletal tongs or halo device.
- NGT for gastric decompression due to paralytic ileus.
- Urinary retention catheter to ↓ bladder distention.
- Multidisciplinary rehabilitation (RT, PT, OT, vocational education).

Nursing Care

- Identify and treat autonomic hyperreflexia: ↑ HOB; loosen clothing; avoid cutaneous stimulation; ensure empty bladder; catheterize to ↓ urinary distention prn; remove fecal mass after application of anesthetic ointment prn.

- Use American Spinal Injury Association (ASIA) scale to determine extent of motor and sensory dysfunction.
- Assess respirations, P, O_2 sat, ABGs; encourage coughing and deep breathing; maintain hydration; provide chest PT.
- Prevent DVT and PE: Assess calf and thigh circumference; give prescribed anticoagulants; use sequential compression devices; avoid popliteal pressure or calf massage.
- ↓ spasticity and prevent contractures: use ROM, splints to ↓ footdrop, trochanter rolls to ↓ external hip rotation; give prescribed antispasmodics.
- Maintain skin integrity: Change position frequently (teach patient to shift weight if able); provide hygiene and massage; provide special bed, mattress, chair cushion; ↑ protein and vitamin C in diet.
- Provide pin site care with halo traction: Cleanse with ordered solution; apply prescribed topical antibiotic.
- Promote fecal elimination: ↑ fluid and fiber intake; assist with bowel training; perform digital stimulation of rectum after meal.
- Promote urinary elimination: Use Credé maneuver; cutaneous stimulus to instigate urination (pull pubic hair, stroke inner thigh); intermittent catheterization if ordered.
- Involve patient with planning; assist with coping with losses; discuss sexual concerns (may have reflex erection and ejaculation).

Gastrointestinal Disorders

Morbid Obesity

- ≥100 lb more than ideal body weight.
- ↑ risk for cardiovascular disease, arthritis, asthma, bronchitis, DM, impaired body image, ↓ self-esteem, depression.

Treatment

- Weight-reduction diet, behavior modification, exercise.
- Bariatric surgery if conservative treatment is unsuccessful (gastric bypass, vertical banded gastroplasty).
- After surgery ↑ risk for peritonitis, obstruction, atelectasis, pneumonia, thromboembolism, nutritional deficiencies, metabolic disturbances due to N&V.
- Antisecretories.

Nursing Care

- Support weight loss, diet modification, exercise regimen.
- **Provide postoperative care**
  - NPO; 6 small feedings daily as ordered (600–800 calories total) when bowel sounds return; ↑ oral fluids to ↓ risk of dehydration.
  - Assess for bleeding, peritonitis, thromboembolism, F&E imbalances.
  - Teach to eat small amounts slowly and chew completely to prevent vomiting and painful esophageal distention.
  - Provide emotional support (body image, dietary restrictions, need for body contouring surgery if desired).

Gastroesophageal Reflux Disease (GERD) and Hiatal Hernia

	Pathophysiology and Etiology	Signs and Symptoms	Treatment
GERD	• Gastric contents enter esophagus, causing inflammation. • May cause a precancerous condition (**Barrett esophagus**). • Related to ↓ tone of lower esophageal sphincter (LES), obesity, hiatal hernia, pregnancy.	• Heartburn (**pyrosis**), hoarseness, wheezing, dysphagia. • Acidic esophageal pH. • Endoscopy or barium swallow reveal tissue damage.	• Meds: Proton pump inhibitors, H_2 receptor blockers, antacids, cholinergics. • Surgery to tighten esophageal fundus.
Hiatal Hernia	• Part of stomach slides upward into thoracic cavity; may cause reflux, obstruction, hemorrhage. • Related to obesity, congenital weakness, pregnancy, female gender.	• May be asymptomatic. • Sense of fullness, regurgitation, pyrosis, dysphagia, nocturnal dyspnea. • Evident in barium swallow.	• Paraesophageal hernias may require emergency surgery to ↓ restricted blood flow. • Meds: See Treatment under GERD.

Nursing Care
• Assess for S&S; support weight control.
• Teach patient to have small, frequent, low-fat meals; drink fluids between meals; remain upright 1 hr after meals.
• Teach patient to ↑ HOB to prevent nighttime distress.
• Advise patient to avoid tight belts and waistbands and to avoid chocolate, caffeine, alcohol, and peppermint, which ↓ LES tone.

Peptic Ulcer Disease and Gastric Carcinoma

Peptic Ulcer Disease (PUD)

Etiology and Pathophysiology	Risk Factors	Signs and Symptoms	Treatment
• ↑ pepsin, ↑ HCl acid or ↓ tissue resistance to acid → gastric or duodenal ulcers. • May → hemorrhage, perforation, or peritonitis.	• *H. pylori*, NSAIDs, alcohol, stress, smoking, Zollinger-Ellison syndrome (↑ HCl).	• Gnawing epigastric pain. • Duodenal ulcer pain occurs 2–3 hr after meals and is relieved by food. • Gastric ulcer pain occurs <1 hr after meals and is relieved by vomiting.	• Proton pump inhibitors, H_2 receptor blockers, antibiotics for *H. pylori*. • Vagotomy to ↓ HCl, antrectomy and reattachment to duodenum (Billroth I) or jejunum (Billroth II).

Gastric Carcinoma

Etiology and Pathophysiology	Risk Factors	Signs and Symptoms	Treatment
• Generally caused by adenocarcinoma, which can metastasize to liver, bone, pancreas, or esophagus before diagnosis.	• Smoked food, pernicious anemia, gastric ulcers, *H. pylori*. • Japanese descent. • Male.	• May be asymptomatic. • Anorexia, ↓ weight, anemia, lack of HCl, heartburn. • Biopsy identifies cancer cells. • Bone and liver scans identify metastasis.	• Gastrectomy, radiation, chemotherapy. • Tumor markers used to check progress (carcinoembryonic antigen, CA19-9, CA50).

Nursing Care

- Assess VS; note amount of coffee ground–like or frank bloody emesis or melena; assess for S&S of shock.
- Manage NG tube and normal saline lavage for bleeding.
- Assess for GI perforation: ↑ P, ↓ BP, abdominal pain, rigid boardlike abdomen, diaphoresis.
- **Dumping syndrome may occur after gastrectomy**
  - Hypertonic gastric contents move rapidly into intestine → shift of intravascular fluid into intestine causing ↓ peripheral vascular resistance, visceral pooling of blood, and reactive hypoglycemia.
  - Results in ↑ P, ↓ BP, diaphoresis, fainting.
  - Limit by teaching no fluid with meals; small, frequent meals; avoid simple carbohydrates; recline 1 hr after meals.

Lower GI Disorders

Inflammatory Bowel Disease (IBD)

Regional Enteritis	Ulcerative Colitis	Diverticulosis and Diverticulitis	Colorectal Cancer
• Crohn disease affects distal ileum and colon. • Mucosal thickening with discrete ulcers. • May → fissures and abscesses that → thick walls and narrow lumen.	• Affects colon and rectum. • Superficial ulcerations cause edema, bleeding; abscesses → thick walls and narrow lumen; ↑ risk of colon cancer.	• Pouchlike herniations in muscle layer of colon (**diverticulosis**). • Trapped food or feces cause inflammation (**diverticulitis**) that may lead to bleeding, obstruction, perforation, and/or peritonitis.	• Adenocarcinoma of epithelial lining invades surrounding tissue by direct extension into lumen → colon narrowing and ulcerations, or metastasis via blood or lymph to other sites (e.g., liver).
• **Risk factors:** Genetics, young adults, smoking.	• **Risk factors:** Jewish, Caucasian, 30–50 yr of age.	• **Risk factors:** ↑ age, genetics, lack of fiber, constipation.	• **Risk factors:** Polyps, IBD, ↑ age, genetics and ↑ fat, ↑ protein, ↓ fiber diet.

	Regional Enteritis	Ulcerative Colitis	Diverticulosis and Diverticulitis	Colorectal Cancer
	• **S&S**: Right lower quadrant (RLQ) cramping pain after meals, ↑T, ↓ weight, diarrhea, rectal bleeding.	• **S&S**: Left lower quadrant (LLQ) abdominal cramps, ↓ weight, rectal bleeding, diarrhea.	• **S&S**: LLQ abdominal pain, ↑T, ↑ WBCs, fatigue, diarrhea or constipation.	• **S&S**: Diarrhea or constipation, ribbon or pencil-shaped stool, ↓ weight, anemia, abdominal distention.
	• **Treatment** • *Meds:* Antidiarrheals, antispasmodics, steroids, metronidazole. • *Exacerbation*: NPO, TPN, intravenous fluid (IVF); then rest bowel with ↓ residue, ↑ protein, ↑ calorie diet. • Colectomy with ileoanal anastomosis, ileostomy, continent ileostomy **(Kock pouch)** if needed. • *Remission:* Maintain balanced diet avoiding foods that aggravate GI mucosa; bulk laxatives to ↓ diarrhea with Chron disease.		• **Treatment** • *Meds:* Antibiotics, antispasmodics. • *Exacerbation:* NPO and then ↓ residue diet until inflammation subsides. • Temporary colostomy or colon resection if needed. • *Remission:* Dietary fiber and bulk laxative to prevent constipation and limit intraluminal intestinal pressure.	• **Treatment** • *Meds:* FOLFOX therapy (5-FU, leucovorin, oxaliplatin [Eloxatin]). • Hemicolectomy or abdominal perineal resection with colostomy, • Radiation, • Monitor carcinoembryonic antigen to mark tumor and response to treatment.

Nursing Care for Patients With Lower GI Disorders

■ Assess for S&S, bowel sounds.
■ Assess for S&S of perforation/peritonitis: Rigid boardlike abdomen, diaphoresis, ↑T, ↑ P, ↓ BP.
■ Assess for shape and consistency of stool; blood in stool **(frank blood, melena)**.
■ Support coping with disease chronicity; teach diet.

- **Provide preoperative care**
  - Provide ordered liquid diet for 48 hr; prescribed antibiotics to ↓ intestinal flora, laxatives and enemas before surgery to empty bowel.
- **Provide postoperative care**
  - Assess VS, breath and bowel sounds; provide pain control; maintain nasogastric decompression until peristalsis resumes, then advance diet as tolerated; teach to avoid gas-forming foods; provide IVs for F&E balance; perform wound care (irrigations or sitz baths for hygiene, comfort, packing removal).
  - Prevent pneumonia: Teach coughing, deep breathing, use of incentive spirometry.
  - Prevent DVT: Teach ankle pumping, early ambulation, apply sequential compression devices, avoid pressure behind the popliteal space.
- **Provide care for the patient with a colostomy**
  - Assess stoma: Pink/brick red is normal; pale, purple, or black indicates ischemia; notify primary health-care provider if stoma is ischemic.
  - Assess bowel sounds, distention, character/amount of stool that usually begins in 3–6 days.
  - Determine consistency of stool; ostomy site determines nature of stool (ileostomy constantly drains liquid stool; sigmoid colostomy stool usually is formed).
  - Apply appliance with 1/8–1/4 inch clearance around stoma to avoid stoma constriction or excess skin exposure to stool.
  - Clean area with soap and water; use prescribed protective barrier and antifungal agent (nystatin) on skin under appliance.
  - Empty appliance when 1/2 full to ↓ leakage.
  - Irrigate distal colostomy with 105°F water at same time daily to regulate elimination.
  - Refer to United Ostomy Association or enterostomal therapist.

Disorders of Accessory Organs of Digestion

Cholecystitis

- Impaired bile flow → gallbladder inflammation (**cholelithiasis**), distention, and autolysis leads to gangrene or perforation; blocked bile flow may → obstructive jaundice.
- Usually due to gallstones or other precipitates.

Risk Factors
- 4 Fs: Fair, Fat, ≥ Forty yr of age, Female.
- Rapid weight loss, estrogen therapy, multiple pregnancies, cirrhosis, DM.

Signs and Symptoms

- RUQ abdominal pain usually radiating to back subscapular area especially after high-fat meal.
- N&V, ↑T, rebound tenderness, obstructive jaundice, yellow skin and sclera, dark urine, clay-colored stools.
- Signs of bleeding due to decreased fat digestion causing ↓ absorption of the fat-soluble vitamin K.
- ↑WBCs, ↑ serum bilirubin, ↑ alkaline phosphatase.

Treatment

- Laparoscopic or abdominal removal of gallbladder **(cholecystectomy)**.
- Incision into common bile duct **(choledochostomy)**.

Nursing Care

- Assess for S&S.
- Teach low-fat diet, use of incentive spirometer, coughing and deep breathing (patient may be reluctant to deep breathe because surgical trauma is near diaphragm).
- Administer prescribed preoperative vitamin K, analgesics.
- Maintain T-tube drainage if bile duct explored; T tube is removed when ductal edema subsides indicated by stool regaining brown color.

Hepatitis

- Inflammation of liver due to infection, parasitic infestation, alcohol, toxins, medications (INH, acetaminophen).
- *Hepatitis A (HAV) and E (HEV):* Spread via fecal-oral route; due to ↓ sanitation and eating shellfish from contaminated water.
- *Hepatitis B (HBV), C (HCV), and D (HDV):* Spread by contact with contaminated blood; due to sexual contact, shared contaminated sharps (needles, razors).

Risk Factors

- Health-care professionals, multiple sexual partners, intravenous drug users.
- Hemophiliacs due to frequent transfusions of clotting factors.
- 30% have unidentifiable sources.

Signs and Symptoms

- May be asymptomatic.
- *Preicteric stage*: Flulike symptoms.
- *Icteric stage:* N&V, anorexia, malaise, jaundice, presence of specific hepatitis antigens and antibodies, ↑ aspartate aminotransferase (AST), ↑ alanine aminotransferase (ALT).

Treatment

- Vaccines against HAV and HBV before exposure provide active immunity.
- Antivirals (interferon); immune globulins provide passive immunity post-exposure.
- Antiretrovirals: Hepatitis B: lamivudine (Epivir-HBV); hepatitis C: Protease inhibitors.

Nursing Care

- Assess for S&S; use contact precautions for HAV and HEV.
- ↑ calories, ↑ protein, ↓ fat in diet as ordered.
- Teach to avoid toxins (acetaminophen, alcohol, carbon tetrachloride, INH).

Cirrhosis

- Fibrous scar tissue and fat accumulate in liver → hepatomegaly and portal hypertension; results in esophageal varices, hemorrhoids, obstructive jaundice, and ascites.
- ↓ liver function → ↓ metabolism → ↑ ammonia (a metabolized protein by-product) → encephalopathy.

Risk Factors

- Alcoholism (most common), hepatitis or biliary disease.
- Industrial chemicals, male gender, 40–60 yr of age.

Signs and Symptoms

- ↑ liver enzymes (AST, ALT, LDH, GGT), jaundice, hepatomegaly.
- ↓ albumin, ↑ bilirubin, ↓ globulins, ↑ ammonia, ↑ prothrombin time.
- Ascites; GI varices; edema due to ↓ albumin and ↑ aldosterone, which causes retention of Na and water.
- Confusion, agitation, flapping hand tremors (**asterixis**).
- Liver biopsy to confirm diagnosis.

Treatment

- Vitamins (A, D, E, K, B), zinc, K-sparing diuretics.
- Lactulose to ↓ ammonia, albumin.
- Portal caval shunt; sclerotherapy or balloon tamponade for varices.
- Paracentesis for ascites with dyspnea.

Nursing Care

- Assess for S&S, I&O, abdominal girth.
- Teach to avoid alcohol if appropriate.
- *Liver biopsy:* Have patient hold breath during needle insertion; keep on right side with pillow against insertion site; assess for bleeding.

- *Paracentesis*: Have patient void before and maintain an upright position during procedure; assess respiratory status, S&S of shock, persistent leakage after procedure.
- *Balloon tamponade*: Provide oral suction; maintain traction on gastric balloon; monitor pressure of esophageal balloon.

Pancreatitis

- Obstruction of pancreatic duct causes reflux of trypsin, resulting in autodigestion of pancreas that leads to inflammation.
- Possible necrosis with calcification, perforation, hemorrhage.
- Pancreatic pseudocysts or abscesses may develop.
- May be idiopathic, acute, or chronic and result in DM.

Risk Factors
- Alcoholism in middle-age men; biliary disease in older females.
- Extremely high triglycerides >1000 mg/dL.

Signs and Symptoms
- Epigastric pain that ↑ with eating and may radiate to thorax/back.
- N&V, ↑T, ↓ weight, abdominal distention, jaundice.
- Steatorrhea and glucose intolerance with chronic pancreatitis.
- ↑ amylase, ↑ lipase, ↓ serum calcium.
- S&S of perforation: Rebound tenderness, rigid abdomen, shock.

Treatment
- NPO; IVF and electrolyte replacement.
- NGT to remove secretions and ↓ GI motility.
- Antibiotics, anticholinergics, pancreatic enzymes (lipase, trypsin, amylase) with meals for chronic pancreatitis.
- Surgery if due to biliary disease.

Nursing Care
- Give prescribed analgesics, antibiotics, anticholinergics, pancreatic enzymes, vitamins A and E.
- Provide diet as ordered (usually low fat); provide small frequent meals.
- Assess I&O; S&S of tetany and hyperglycemia.
- Support abstinence from alcohol; refer to Alcoholics Anonymous if appropriate.

Nursing Care for Patients Receiving Nutritional Support

Parenteral Nutrition (PN)

Introduction

- Nutrients are administered directly into bloodstream, bypassing the GI tract.
- For patients who are unable to absorb nutrients or have high nutritive demands (severe burns, cancer, multiple trauma, cancer); rests GI tract.
- PN solutions are hypertonic and formulated to meet individual needs; include amino acids, glucose, vitamins, minerals, trace elements, heparin, insulin; lipid emulsions containing essential fatty acids, triglycerides, and supplemental kilocalories may be given weekly.
- Catheter is advanced to superior vena cava to promote dilution of formula and prevent intima inflammation.
- **Total parenteral nutrition (TPN):** Catheter inserted into subclavian or jugular vein and advanced to superior vena cava; used when PN is required for a long period of time.
- **Partial parenteral nutrition (PPN):** Peripherally inserted central catheter (PICC); inserted into vein of arm and advanced to superior vena cava; used when PN is required for a short period of time or to supplement oral nutrition.

Nursing Care for Patients Receiving Parenteral Nutrition

- Ensure catheter placement is radiographically confirmed before use.
- Verify order for formula, amount, and rate of infusion; verify expiration date on formula; label solution bag with date, time, and formula type.
- Use an infusion pump; dedicate a port to prevent interactions with IVF or IV medications.
- Keep PN solution refrigerated; return to room temperature naturally because cold solution can cause pain, venous spasm, and hypothermia.
- Infuse slowly initially; ↑ rate in increments of 25 mL/hr until ordered rate is reached; maintain consistent rate.
- Monitor for metabolic and F&E imbalances because they may indicate intolerance; may need to ↓ rate or halt flow until problem is corrected.
- Monitor blood glucose every 6 hr because PN solutions are high in glucose; administer insulin coverage as ordered.

- **Prevent infection**
  - Use meticulous sterile technique when changing transparent occlusive dressing over insertion site every 72 hr; cleanse port before/after use with 70% alcohol or chlorhexidine gluconate-based pads.
  - Change infusion sets every 24 hr; ensure tubing has an in-line filter for PN; use set specific for lipids and use port below PN filter if being given concurrently.
  - Discard unused solution after 24 hr; avoid using if a leak, cloudiness, or floating particles are identified.
  - Progressively wean off PN to ↓ risk of metabolic problems (over 48 hr); if abrupt discontinuation of PN is necessary give a 5% or 10% dextrose solution to prevent rebound hypoglycemia until primary health-care provider is notified.
- **Monitor for complications and notify health-care provider if one occurs**
  - *Pneumothorax:* Puncture of lung during catheter insertion allows air in pleural cavity. S&S: Severe sudden chest pain, marked dyspnea, absent breath sounds on affected side. Nursing care: Elevate HOB, administer oxygen, monitor VS and oxygen saturation, assist with chest tube insertion.
  - Catheter occlusion: Debris or blood clot at tip of catheter. S&S: Sluggish or absent catheter flow rate. Nursing care: Stop infusion; follow protocol such as flush with heparin or saline, aspirate clot, use thrombolytic agent.
  - *Infection:* Pathogens enter blood via catheter or insertion site. S&S: ↑VS, chills, positive blood culture. Nursing care: Administer local and/or systemic antibiotics and antipyretics.
  - *Hyperglycemia:* SNS stimulation of stress hormones and high glucose load of solution ↑serum glucose level. S&S: Polyuria, polydipsia, headache, lethargy, increased serum glucose level. Nursing care: Administer insulin coverage as prescribed.
- Document patient response, I&O, weekly weight (should gain about 3 lb).

Enteral Nutrition (Tube Feeding)

Introduction
- Liquid formula administered via tube into stomach or jejunum.
- For patients with intact GI systems but who have impaired swallowing, high nutritive demands, or are unable to meet nutritional needs orally.
- Tube advanced through nose into stomach (nasogastric [NG] tube), abdominal wall into stomach (percutaneous endoscopic gastrostomy [PEG] tube), or abdominal wall into jejunum (jejunostomy tube [J-tube]).

- Standard formulas balanced with 12%–20% protein, 45%–60% carbohy-drates, 30%–40% fats, vitamins and minerals; specialty formulas such as high protein, high fiber, renal, pulmonary, and hydrolyzed formulas are used for specific health problems.
- Feedings may be continuous, intermittent (bolus), or cyclical (continuous feeding administered for less than 24 hr a day).

Nursing Care for Patients Receiving a Tube Feeding

- Confirm tube placement: radiographically before first use; before each use or every 4 hr for continuous/cyclical feedings via NG or PEG tube; use several methods.
  - Aspirate stomach contents: pH is normally acidic (1.5–3.5) greenish/yellow color; residual gastric volume should not exceed parameter such as >½ previous feeding; if excessive, hold feeding 1 hr and reassess; reinstill aspirate to prevent electrolyte and acid/base imbalances.
  - Instill 10–30 mL of air in tube while auscultating epigastric area; "whoosh" sound with gurgling is heard as air enters stomach.
- Secure NG tube to naris and assess naris skin every 4 hr; change sterile dressing to PEG or J-tube site every 8 hr until healed and then provide meticulous skin care.
- Verify order for formula, amount, and rate of infusion; verify expiration date on formula; label solution bag with date, time, and formula type.
- Wash hands; don clean gloves; raise HOB throughout feeding and 1 hr after bolus feeding; assess placement; measure and assess aspirate; flush tube with 30 mL water; instill bolus feeding or begin continuous/cyclical feeding; flush tube with 30 mL of water after bolus feeding or routinely with continuous/cyclical feeding; instill additional water as ordered.
- **Monitor for complications and notify primary health-care provider if one occurs.**
  - *Aspiration:* Gastric contents enter respiratory tract due to gastric reflux or vomiting. S&S: Coughing, SOB, dyspnea, restlessness, ↑ P, ↑ R, ↓ O$_2$ sat. Nursing Care: Elevate HOB, administer oxygen, suction airway.
  - *Diarrhea:* Liquid stool due to hyperosmolar formula, rapid administration, malabsorption, cold formula, tube migration from stomach into small intestine, bacterial contamination. S&S: Frequent unformed stools, abdominal cramping. Nursing care: assess bowel sounds and amount and character of stool, give prescribed antidiarrheal or probiotic such as *L. acidophilus.*
  - *Dumping syndrome:* hypertonic solution rapidly enters intestine pulling fluid from intestinal wall into lumen. S&S: ↑peristalsis, ↑bowel sounds, abdominal pain, vomiting, and release of insulin in relation to hyper-glycemia ultimately causing weakness, shakiness, anxiety, sweating, ↑ P,

confusion. Nursing care: halt infusion, obtain order for slower rate or different formula, encourage rest/reclining position after a feeding.

- *Tube obstruction:* Occurs when tube is inadequately flushed, medications are inadequately crushed, a feeding is on hold to provide nursing care, a feeding *runs dry*. S&S: Slow or absent flow rate; Nursing Care: ensure tube is not compressed or has dependent loops, reposition patient with instructions to cough, flush tube with water or cranberry juice.

■ Document patient response, I&O, weekly weight (should gain about 3 lb).

Female Reproductive Cancers

Breast Cancer

■ Development of malignant cells due to hormonal, genetic, and/or environmental factors.
■ Localized or invasive; may affect lobules (lobular carcinoma) or ducts (ductal carcinoma [Paget disease]).
■ Stage 0 (in situ), Stage 1 (tumor <2 cm), Stage 2 (tumor 2–5 cm), Stage 3 (tumor >5 cm), Stage 4 (metastasis).

Risk Factors
■ ↑ age, female gender, family history, *BRCA-1* and *BRCA-2* genes.
■ Nulliparity or late first pregnancy, estrogen replacement, early menarche, late menopause.
■ Alcohol, obesity, cancer in other breast.

Signs and Symptoms
■ Hard, nontender mass; often superior lateral breast; may attach to underlying tissue (fixed).
■ Recent inversion or flattening of nipple; itchy, scaly nipple lesion.
■ Unilateral venous prominence.
■ Orange peel appearance of breast tissue (**peau d'orange**).
■ Enlarged axillary nodes.
■ Diagnostic tests: Mammogram; sonogram; MRI; estrogen receptor and progesterone receptor assays to determine tumor's sensitivity to hormones; scans and tumor markers (Ca 15–3, Ca 125, carcinoembryonic antigen) to determine progression; tumor biopsy.
■ Sentinel node biopsy identifies primary axillary node for breast drainage and need for standard vs. invasive axillary node dissection.

Treatment
■ Based on stage: Lumpectomy, mastectomy, nodal dissection, radiation, chemotherapy, hormonal therapy, bone marrow transplantation.

- Reconstruction surgery may involve progressive addition of saline into temporary implants to expand tissue before insertion of final implants; patient's own muscle flaps from abdomen or back are used to simulate breast tissue; tissue from inner thigh or labia is used to create nipple; tattoo to simulate areola.

Nursing Care

- Assess for S&S.
- **Teach monthly breast self-examination (BSE)**
  - Systematic light, medium, and deep palpation with finger pads over breasts and axilla once a month.
  - 5–7 days after start of menses in premenopausal women and same day every month in postmenopausal women.
  - Inspect for symmetry, dimpling, or nipple inversion.
- **Provide care for patient receiving radiation**
  - Balance rest/activity to manage fatigue.
  - Prevent irritating site: Avoid sun, wearing bras, using ointments, lotions, or powders; wear soft cotton clothing.
- **Provide care during postoperative period**
  - Provide for pain management.
  - Maintain portable wound drainage device to ↓ edema.
  - Teach postmastectomy exercises (wall climbing) to ↑ muscle strength, ↑ contractures; ↓ risk of lymphedema.
  - Protect upper extremity on side of surgery; No BPs, IVs, injections, or withdrawal of blood specimens; teach patient to avoid lifting or carrying heavy items, use electric razor for axillary hair, wear gloves for gardening.
  - Provide support of patient and partner; refer to Reach to Recovery.
  - Provide care for patient receiving antineoplastic medications (see Nursing Care for Patients With Cancer or Experiencing Nontherapeutic Effects of Antineoplastic Therapies, p. 178).

Cervical Cancer

- 90% from squamous cells; 10% adenocarcinoma.
- High cure rate if diagnosed in situ.

Risk Factors

- 30–45 yr of age, human papillomavirus, sexual activity at young age, multiple sex partners, HIV.

Signs and Symptoms

- Early: Watery vaginal secretion initially progressing to foul-smelling discharge, bleeding between menses (**metrorrhagia**) or after intercourse; positive Pap smear.
- Late: Back and leg pain, leg edema, dysuria, rectal bleeding, anemia, ↑ weight.

Treatment
- Based on stage, cryotherapy or laser therapy, removal of part of cervix that maintains reproductive function (**conization**), hysterectomy, loop electro-cautery excision procedure.
- External radiation; intracavity radiation (**brachytherapy**).

Nursing Care
- Provide emotional support.
- **Provide care for patient receiving external radiation**
  - Assess for skin lesion, nausea, diarrhea, cystitis, fistulas.
  - Encourage patient to wear soft cotton underwear, avoid nylon underwear and pantyhose.
  - Teach patient perineal care.
- **Provide care for patient receiving internal radiation**
  - Pregnant nurses must not care for patients receiving internal radiation.
  - Provide private room; consider time/distance/shielding; organize care to ↓ time in room.
  - Prevent dislodgment of intracavity device: Maintain supine position (usually 1–3 days); indwelling urinary catheter; low-residue diet and antidiarrheals.
- **Provide postoperative care**
  - Assess for bleeding and infection; provide pain management; encourage use of incentive spirometer; teach DVT prevention such as ankle-pumping exercises, compression device.
  - Provide care for patient receiving antineoplastic medications (see Nursing Care for Patients With Cancer or Experiencing Nontherapeutic Effects of Antineoplastic Therapies, p. 178)

Ovarian Cancer

- 90% epithelial in origin.
- Lower incidence than other GYN cancers but ↑ mortality since most metastasize before diagnosis.

Risk Factors
- Breast cancer; *BRCA-1* and *BRCA-2* genes; Caucasians (lowest for Asians).
- Industrialized society, high-fat diet, oral contraceptives, nulliparity, multipara.

Signs and Symptoms
- May be asymptomatic until advanced.
- Enlarged ovary on palpation; ↑ abdominal girth due to tumor or ascites.
- Anemia; ↓ weight; constipation; flatulence; urinary frequency; leg or pelvic pain.
- ↑ Ca-125 tumor antigen; tumor seen on transvaginal ultrasound.

Treatment

■ Total abdominal hysterectomy: Uterus, ovaries, fallopian tubes, omentum.
■ Chemotherapy with cyclophosphamide, doxorubicin, cisplatin.
■ Ca-125 levels to assess progress.
■ Paracentesis for palliation.

Nursing Care

■ Provide emotional support.
■ **Provide postoperative care**
  ■ Assess for bleeding and infection.
  ■ Provide for pain management.
  ■ Encourage incentive spirometry; implement DVT prevention.
  ■ Provide care for patient receiving antineoplastic therapy (see Nursing Care for Patients With Cancer or Experiencing Nontherapeutic Effects of Antineoplastic Therapies, p. 178).

Infectious Diseases

Lyme Disease and Tetanus

	Lyme Disease	Tetanus (Lockjaw)
Etiology and Pathophysiology	• *Borrelia burgdorferi:* Spirochete; infected deer or mouse → tick → human through tick's bite. • 3–30 day incubation.	• *Clostridium tetani:* Anaerobic bacillus; enters puncture wound, resulting in bacterial toxins affecting nervous system → muscle spasms. • 3–21 day incubation.
Risk Factors	• Northeastern United States, wooded areas.	• No tetanus toxoid to produce active immunity.
S&S	• Early: Bull's-eye rash. • Later: Arthritis, Bell palsy, meningitis, carditis, dementia, paralysis.	• Spasms of voluntary muscles causing pain, abnormal postures, and facial expressions. • Respiratory spasm and failure.
Treatment	• Amoxicillin, doxycycline, ceftriaxone.	• Tetanus immune globulin, supportive care.

	Lyme Disease	**Tetanus (Lockjaw)**
Nursing Care	• Provide supportive care. • Teach to complete antibiotic therapy; wear long, light-colored clothes to see ticks; avoid tall grass; use bug repellent; inspect skin; use tweezers to remove tick.	• Maintain airway. • Immune globulin for brief passive immunity. • Wound care. • Teach need for tetanus toxoid boosters every 10 yr for active immunity.

HIV and AIDS

■ Acquired immunodeficiency syndrome (AIDS) caused by human immunodeficiency virus (HIV).

■ HIV infects helper T lymphocytes (T4/CD4 cells), B lymphocytes, macrophages, promyelocytes, fibroblasts.

■ Opportunistic infections occur when T4/CD4 cell count <200/µL (*Pneumocystis jiroveci* pneumonia, histoplasmosis, *Mycobacterium tuberculosis*, cytomegalovirus).

■ HIV transmitted through contact with infected body fluids (blood, semen, vaginal secretions, blood-tinged saliva, tears, breast milk, cerebrospinal fluid).

■ Incubation period is 6 months–10 yr or longer; tests can detect virus within 24 hr; antibodies detected within 2–36 months or longer.

Signs and symptoms

■ Anorexia, fatigue, chills, sore throat, dyspnea, night sweats, lymphadenopathy.

■ Weight loss of 10% or more, constant fever, chronic diarrhea and weakness **(wasting syndrome)**.

■ Memory loss, ↓ cognition, ↓ coordination, partial paralysis **(HIV encephalopathy)**.

■ Presence of opportunistic infections and malignancies such as Kaposi sarcoma.

■ Enzyme-linked immunosorbent assay (ELISA) test for screening; Western blot to confirm positive ELISA; polymerase chain reaction for presence of HIV; HIV RNA for evidence of viral load.

Treatment

- Highly active antiretroviral therapy (HAART); three or more drugs from at least two classes of drugs that ↓ HIV replication; fusion inhibitor; integrase inhibitors; protease inhibitors (PIs); non-nucleoside reverse transcriptase inhibitors (NNRTIs); nucleoside reverse transcriptase inhibitors (NRTIs); antivirals (See Tab 7, MEDS, Antiretrovirals, p. 257)
- Medications to treat opportunistic infections such as TB.
- NRTIs for postexposure prophylaxis (PEP) such as after accidental needle sticks.

Nursing Care

- Assess for S&S; VS, weight loss; progression of clinical manifestations; S&S of opportunistic infections.
- Maintain standard precautions; institute transmission based precautions for patient with opportunistic infections.
- Encourage verbalization of feelings; explain chronicity of condition.
- Encourage adherence to medication regimen because nonadherence leads to resistant strains; assess for and teach patient common side effects (see Tab 7, MEDS, Antiretrovirals, p. 257).
- Teach patient to inform sexual contacts of diagnosis; use safer sex (condom with water-soluble jelly); avoid breastfeeding and sharing needles.
- Teach patient to protect self from infection: Avoid crowds, undercooked meats, small animals; perform hand hygiene often.
- Encourage ↑ calorie, ↑ protein diet with foods high in immune-stimulating nutrients such as vitamins A, C, and E, and selenium.

Perioperative Nursing Care

Preoperative Nursing Care

Identify Physical and Emotional Risk Factors

- *Cardiopulmonary status:* RBCs, WBCs, Hb, Hct, chest x-ray, ECG (over 40 yr of age or preexisting condition).
- *Bleeding/clotting risk:* Platelets, PT, PTT, INR, type and cross for blood transfusion.
- *Identification of preexisting conditions:* BUN and creatinine (kidney function); liver enzymes (liver function); fasting blood glucose (DM); hCG (pregnancy).
- *Emotional status:* Assess for positive or negative attitude regarding surgery and expected outcome; inform surgeon if patient has an attitude of impending doom.

Provide Teaching

- *Expectations:* Such as pain management plan,
- *Skills:* Leg exercises, diaphragmatic breathing, coughing, use of incentive spirometer.
- *Care related to specific surgeries:* See specific diseases.

Preparation of Patient on Day of Surgery

- *Secure informed consent:* Surgeon explains surgery/risks; nurse witnesses patient's signature.
- *Prevent aspiration:* Restriction of oral intake; give prescribed anticholinergic to ↓ respiratory secretions; H_2 receptor antagonist to ↓ gastric acid.
- *Prevent surgical site infection:* Cleanse skin with ordered antimicrobial agent such as chlorhexidine.
- *Limit anxiety and maximize anesthetic agent:* Give prescribed CNS depressant such as a sedative or opioid.
- *Implement "time-out" huddle:* Verify patient name, type of surgery, site; ensure OR checklist is complete.

Intraoperative Nursing Care

Role of nurse

- *Circulating nurse:* Coordinates environment/practices to ensure patient safety; positions patient with anesthesiologist to promote access to surgical site while maintaining functional alignment; ensures grounding of patient and equipment; participates in "time-out" huddle to verify patient, surgery, and site.
- *Scrub person:* Prepares surgical equipment, assists surgeon, ensures patient safety such as performs instrument count.

Postoperative Nursing Care

- *Maintain airway*
  - Assess VS, oxygen saturation, sputum characteristics, breath sounds (for atelectasis or pneumonia.
  - Administer oxygen, remove artificial airway when gag reflex returns, suction airway if necessary, position on side if vomiting.
  - Encourage coughing and deep breathing (splint incision), use of incentive spirometer.
- *Maintain portable wound drainage devices*
  - Empty and recompress self-contained suction devices (Hemovac, Jackson Pratt) when half full of drainage to reestablish negative pressure.
  - Ensure patency, avoid dependent loops, assess amount and characteristics of drainage.

- *Manage pain*
  - Assess location, characteristics, and extent of pain (use pain rating scale).
  - Give prescribed analgesic (usually IV via patient-controlled analgesia [PCA]).
  - Use nonpharmacological interventions (imagery, relaxation exercises).
- *Assess for S&S of hypovolemic shock due to hemorrhage*
  - Bloody drainage; weak, rapid pulse; ↑ R; ↓ BP; ↓ urine output (<30 mL/hr); ↓ Hb; ↓ Hct.
  - Pallor; cold, clammy skin; maintain intravascular volume (administer ordered transfusions, IVFs).
- *Assess for and prevent neurovascular complications*
  - Assess for unilateral leg edema, inflammation, calf pain caused by dorsiflexion of foot (Homan sign) that may indicate thrombophlebitis; do not elicit Homan sign because it may cause a thrombus to become an embolus.
  - Assess for sudden chest pain, SOB, ↓ Sao₂ that may indicate PE.
  - Encourage early ambulation, leg exercises, use of sequential compression devices, ↑ fluids.
  - Avoid popliteal pressure; give prophylactic anticoagulants.
  - Assess peripheral neurovascular status after spinal anesthesia or extremity surgery such as peripheral pulse, capillary refill, color and temperature of skin, sensation, and mobility of distal extremity.
- *Prevent urinary retention*
  - Assess for inability to void, voiding small amounts often, suprapubic distention.
  - Encourage frequent position change; ↑ fluids; may need to secure order to catheterize.
- *Prevent paralytic (postoperative) ileus*
  - Assess for absence of bowel sounds, abdominal distention, vomiting.
  - Maintain nasogastric tube to suction for decompression; assess amount and characteristics of drainage.
  - Encourage early ambulation, fluids, dietary fiber as ordered.
- *Identify wound complications*
  - Provide food ↑ in vitamin C and protein within dietary order to facilitate wound healing.
  - Prevent tension on incision such as splinting, abdominal binders, antiemetic to prevent vomiting.
  - Assess approximation of wound edges especially between the 5th to 10th postoperative days; separation of wound edges (**dehiscence**); protrusion of internal organs through incision (**evisceration**); associated with obesity, coughing and straining; evisceration requires emergency care such as low-Fowler position, application of sterile moist saline dressing, notification of surgeon.
  - Assess for S&S of infection such as inflammation, purulent exudate, ↑T; use surgical asepsis for wound care; implement contact precautions.

Common Therapeutic Drug Classifications
    Antacids
    Antidiarrheals
    Antibiotics and Anti-infectives
    Anticoagulants
    Antiemetics
    Antifungals
    Antiparasitics
    Analgesics, Antipyretics, NSAIDs
    Antihistamines
    Antihypertensives
    Antilipidemics (Lipid Lowering)
    Antineoplastics and Related Medications
    Antituberculars
    Antiretrovirals
    Antivirals
    Bronchodilators
    Antisecretory Agents
    Diuretics
    Thrombolytic Agents
    Hypoglycemics (Oral)
    Insulins
    Laxatives and Cathartics
    Opioid (Narcotic) Antagonists
    Opioid (Narcotic) Analgesics
    Opioid and Nonopioid Analgesic Combinations
    Antiseizure Agents
    Bone Resorption Inhibitors
Obstetric Medications
Hormonal Disorders and Related Medications
    Hyperthyroidism
    Hypothyroidism
    Hyperparathyroidism
    Diabetes Insipidus
    Cushing Syndrome
    Addison Disease
    Hyperpituitarism
    Premature Menopause and Menopausal Symptoms
    Erectile Dysfunction
    Contraception
    Emergency Contraception
    Prostate Cancer

Common Therapeutic Drug Classifications

Antacids: Decrease Gastric Acidity and Epigastric Pain and Protect Stomach Mucosa

Mechanism of Action	Examples	Nontherapeutic Effects
Bind with excess acid.	aluminum hydroxide (Amphojel) magnesium/aluminum hydroxide (Maalox, Mylanta)	• Aluminum salts ↓ stool transit causing constipation, hypophosphatemia. • Magnesium salts ↑ peristalsis causing diarrhea, hypermagnesemia.

Nursing Care
- Many antacids contain Na, which should be avoided on low Na diets.
- Shake suspensions well; give 60 mL water to ↑ passage to stomach.
- Encourage foods high in calcium and iron; avoid foods that ↑ GI distress.
- Caution about overuse, which may cause alkalosis, rebound hyperacidity.
- Assess for extent and relief of epigastric and abdominal pain.
- Assess emesis and stool for frank and occult blood.
- Teach to report signs and symptoms (S&S) if they do not resolve in 2 weeks.
- Monitor serum calcium and phosphate levels with chronic use.

Antidiarrheals: Decrease Diarrhea and Promote Formed Stool

Mechanism of Action	Examples	Nontherapeutic Effects
Motility suppressants ↓ peristalsis so water is absorbed by large intestine.	diphenoxylate (Lomotil) loperamide (Imodium)	Tachycardia, respiratory depression, ileus, urinary retention, sedation, dry mouth.
Enteric bacteria replacements ↓ pathogenic bacterial growth.	*lactobacillus acidophilus* (Bacid)	Abdominal cramps, ↑ flatulence.

Nursing Care

- Assess bowel movements for frequency, characteristics; assess bowel sounds for ↓ in hyperactivity.
- Assess for fluid and electrolyte (F&E) imbalances, particularly dehydration.

Antibiotics and Anti-infectives Destroy or Decrease Growth of Susceptible Microorganisms

Mechanism of Action	Examples	Nontherapeutic Effects
Aminoglycosides ↓ protein synthesis.	gentamicin neomycin	• Nausea and vomiting (N&V), hyper-sensitivity reactions such as rash and anaphylaxis.
Cephalosporins Bind to cell wall, causing cell death.	cefazolin (Ancef) ceftriaxone (Rocephin) cephalexin (Keflex)	
Fluoroquinolones ↓ DNA synthesis.	levofloxacin (Levaquin) ciprofloxacin (Cipro)	
Macrolides ↓ protein synthesis.	azithromycin (Zithromax) clarithromycin (Biaxin)	
Penicillins Bind to cell wall → cell death.	amoxicillin penicillin V	
Sulfonamides ↓ protein synthesis.	doxycycline (Vibramycin) tetracycline (Sumycin)	
Anti-infectives ↓ protein and DNA synthesis; bactericidal, trichomonacidal, amebicidal.	chloroquine phosphate (Aralen) metronidazole (Flagyl)	

Nursing Care

- Ensure culture and sensitivity (C&S) test is done before starting medication; assess S&S of hepatotoxicity, nephrotoxicity, hyperglycemia, drug interactions associated with some fluoroquinolones.
- Assess S&S of infection.
- Assess for superinfection: Furry overgrowth on tongue; vaginal discharge; foul-smelling stools.

- Give evenly spaced doses to maintain blood levels.
- Teach regimen should be completed to prevent resistance.
- Do not crush or chew extended-release tablets.
- Obtain blood specimen 1–3 hr after a dose (depending on medication) to measure highest blood level (**peak**) and 30–60 min before next dose to measure lowest blood level (**trough**).

Anticoagulants: Interfere With Normal Coagulation to Decrease Thrombus Formation or Extension

Mechanism of Action	Examples	Nontherapeutic Effects
Thrombin inhibitors ↓ conversion of prothrombin to thrombin, thus ↓ conversion of fibrinogen to fibrin.	heparin lepirudin (Refludan)	• Excessive bleeding such as bruising, melena, hematuria, epistaxis, bleeding gums. • ↓ hemoglobin (Hb) and ↓ hematocrit (Hct), anemia, thrombocytopenia.
Low molecular weight heparins Block coagulation factor Xa.	dalteparin (Fragmin) enoxaparin (Lovenox) rivaroxaban (Xarelto)	
Clotting factor inhibitors Interfere with hepatic synthesis of vitamin K and dependent clotting factors.	warfarin (Coumadin)	
Platelet inhibitors ↓ platelet aggregation.	clopidogrel (Plavix) ticlopidine (Ticlid) aspirin	
Direct thrombin inhibitor Attaches to thrombin ↓ its ability to clot.	dabigatran (Pradaxa)	• Same as above. • Dyspepsia, esophagitis. • Hypersensitivity reactions.

Nursing Care

- Discontinue anticoagulants before invasive procedures; report if bleeding occurs; prepare to give antidote (protamine sulfate for heparin, vitamin K for warfarin); encourage use of medical alert card or jewelry.
- Assess for bleeding; monitor coagulation studies, platelet count; use electric razor, soft toothbrush; teach to avoid over-the-counter (OTC) medications, especially aspirin and NSAIDs.
- Avoid alcohol and foods high in vitamin K, as they ↓ medication effectiveness.
- *Thrombin inhibitors:* Monitor partial thromboplastin time (PTT—therapeutic level is 1.5–2.5 times control); half-life of heparin is 1–2 hr.
- *Low molecular weight heparins:* Do not use with another heparin product; if bruising occurs, ice cube massage site before injection.
- *Clotting factor inhibitors:* Monitor prothrombin time (PT—therapeutic level is 1.3–2.0 times control) or international normalized ratio (INR—therapeutic level is 2–4.5 times control).

Antiemetics Decrease N&V and Prevent and Decrease Motion Sickness

Mechanism of Action	Examples	Nontherapeutic Effects
Phenothiazines ↓ chemoreceptor trigger zone in central nervous system (CNS).	prochlorperazine (Compazine) promethazine (Phenergan)	Confusion, sedation, photosensitivity, dry mouth, constipation, extrapyramidal reactions.
5 HT$_3$ antagonists Block serotonin at receptor sites in vagal nerve terminals and chemoreceptor trigger zone in CNS.	ondansetron (Zofran)	Headache, dizziness, constipation, diarrhea.
Anticholinergics Correct imbalance of acetylcholine and norepinephrine in CNS that causes motion sickness.	scopolamine (Transderm Scop) trimethobenzamide (Tigan)	• Drowsiness. • *Scopolamine:* Urinary hesitancy, blurred vision, dry mouth, tachycardia. • *Tigan suppository:* ↓ blood pressure (BP), local irritation.

Mechanism of Action	Examples	Nontherapeutic Effects
Nonphenothiazines Block chemoreceptor trigger zone in CNS; ↑ gastrointestinal (GI) motility and ↑ gastric emptying.	metoclopramide (Reglan)	Extrapyramidal reactions, restlessness, drowsiness, anxiety, depression.

Nursing Care

- Give 30–60 min before chemotherapy or activity that causes motion sickness.
- Assess vital signs (VS); extent and relief of N&V; abdominal distention.
- Ensure safety because of CNS depression; avoid alcohol and other CNS depressants.
- *Assess for extrapyramidal reactions:* Involuntary movements, grimacing, rigidity, shuffling gait, trembling.
- *Phenothiazines:* Encourage sunscreen and protective clothing; assess for **neuroleptic malignant syndrome:** Hyperthermia, diaphoresis, unstable BP, dyspnea, stupor, muscle rigidity, urinary incontinence.

Antifungals: Decrease Fungal Growth

Mechanism of Action	Examples	Nontherapeutic Effects
Systemic antifungals Impair fungal plasma membrane.	clotrimazole (Mycelex) fluconazole (Diflucan) nystatin (Mycostatin)	• Teratogenic, F&E imbalance, N&V, diarrhea, rash, fever. • Nephrotoxicity, ototoxicity, and hepatotoxicity.
Topical antifungals Disrupt fungal cell wall and metabolism.	amphotericin B (Fungizone) clotrimazole ketoconazole (Nizoral) nystatin (Mycostatin)	Burning, irritation.

Nursing Care

- *Systemic:* Assess for nephrotoxicity, hepatotoxicity, ototoxicity.
- Complete entire regimen; prevent pregnancy; assess for hypoglycemia in patient with diabetes mellitus (DM).
- *Topical:* Assess for irritation; clean skin with tepid water before application.
- Teach difference between *swish and swallow* and *swish and spit*.
- Teach how to administer a vaginal medication and to abstain from intercourse until infection clears.

Antiparasitics: Cause Parasite Death

Mechanism of Action	Examples	Nontherapeutic Effects
Parasiticidal Directly absorbed into parasites and eggs (scabies, lice).	lindane	CNS toxicity, seizures.
	permethrin (Nix)	Pruritus, tingling.
Anthelmintic Prevents pinworm growth and reproduction.	mebendazole (Vermox)	• Hypersensitivity such as rash, anaphylaxis. • Abdominal pain.

Nursing Care

- Maintain standard precautions.
- Teach to wash bedding, clothes, etc., in hot water and dryer; vacuum carpets and furniture; seal nonwashables in plastic bags for 2 weeks; teach hand hygiene before meals and after toileting; treat all family members.
- *Pediculosis/scabies:* Use contact precautions and hair cap with direct care; scrub body with soap and water, dry, apply medication while avoiding wounds, mucous membranes, face, eyes.
- *Pinworms:* Collect specimen with cellophane tape test in a.m.; assess perianal area.
- *Head lice:* Shampoo for 5 min; use fine-tooth comb to remove eggs (nits).

Analgesics, Antipyretics, and NSAIDs Decrease Pain, Fever, and Inflammation

Mechanism of Action	Examples	Nontherapeutic Effects
Analgesic only Inhibit prostaglandins involved in pain or fever.	acetaminophen (Tylenol)	Hepatic toxicity.
Nonsalicylate NSAID Inhibit prostaglandins involved in fever, inflammation, pain.	ibuprofen (Advil, Motrin) naproxen (Aleve, Naprosyn)	Rash, tinnitus, flulike syndrome.
Salicylates NSAID Inhibit prostaglandins involved in inflammation, pain, fever.	acetylsalicylic acid (aspirin, Ecotrin)	• Agitation, hyperventilation, lethargy, confusion, diarrhea. • *Toxicity:* Diaphoresis, tinnitus (8th cranial nerve damage).

Nursing Care

- Do not exceed recommended 24-hr dose; withhold 1 week before invasive procedures because of ↓ platelet aggregation and risk of bleeding; salicylates contraindicated in pregnancy, lactation, children <2 yrs of age (associated with Reye syndrome).
- Give with 8 ounces (oz) water, sit up 15–30 min after ingestion; give with food except for naproxen and ibuprofen; assess for GI bleeding (anemia, melena).
- Avoid alcohol and OTC drugs with analgesic or antipyretic properties.
- Discontinue medication and report serious side effects.
- *Acetaminophen:* Do not exceed >4 g per 24-hr period to ↓ risk of hepatotoxicity.
- *Salicylates:* Monitor serum salicylate levels.
- *NSAIDs:* Assess for headache, drowsiness, dizziness, photosensitivity.

Antihistamines Decrease Clinical Indicators of Allergies and Motion Sickness

Mechanism of Action	Examples	Nontherapeutic Effects
Block histamine, which ↓ allergic response and motion sickness.	diphenhydramine (Benadryl) loratadine (Claritin)	Dry eyes and mouth, constipation, blurred vision, sedation.

Nursing Care

- Contraindicated with narrow-angle glaucoma; use caution with opioids because it may cause paradoxical effect.
- May be used to promote sleep; assess older adults for risk of falls.
- Exerts antiemetic, anticholinergic, CNS depressant effects; assess older adults for confusion.
- Give with food and fluid to ↓ GI irritation.
- Caution patient to avoid hazardous activities; assess level of sedation.
- Give 1 hr before activity for motion sickness prophylaxis.
- Suggest use of gum and hard candy to ↑ salivation and ↑ dry mouth.
- Teach to wear long sleeves and pants and sunscreen.

Antihypertensives: Decrease Blood Pressure (also see Diuretics, p. 262)

Mechanism of Action	Examples	Nontherapeutic Effects
Angiotensin antagonists (ACE inhibitors) ↓ release of aldosterone causing ↑ excretion of Na and water.	enalapril (Vasotec) fosinopril (Monopril) lisinopril (Prinivil, Zestril) ramipril (Altace)	Teratogenic, cough, taste disturbances, proteinuria, agranulocytosis, angioedema, neutropenia.

Mechanism of Action	Examples	Nontherapeutic Effects
Calcium channel blockers ↑ relaxation and dilation of vascular smooth muscle of coronary arteries and arterioles.	amlodipine (Norvasc) diltiazem (Cardizem) nifedipine (Procardia) verapamil (Calan)	• Flushing, peripheral edema. • *Cardizem, Calan:* Bradycardia.
Angiotensin II receptor antagonists ↓ vasoconstriction and ↓ release of aldosterone.	irbesartan (Avapro) losartan (Cozaar) valsartan (Diovan)	• Teratogenic, nephrotoxic. • May cause angioedema such as dyspnea, facial swelling.
Beta blockers (selective) Block stimulation of beta₁ (myocardial) adrenergic receptors.	metoprolol (Lopressor)	• Fatigue, weakness, impotence, bradycardia, pulmonary edema. • May ↑ blood glucose of patients with DM.
Beta blockers (nonselective) Block stimulation of beta₁ (myocardial) and beta₂ (pulmonary, vascular, uterine) adrenergic receptors.	carvedilol (Coreg) labetalol (Normodyne) propranolol (Inderal)	• Fatigue, weakness, pulmonary edema, bradycardia. • May cause impotence.
Centrally acting antiadrenergics Stimulate CNS alpha₂ adrenergic receptors to ↓ sympathetic outflow.	clonidine (Catapres) methyldopa (Aldomet)	• Dizziness, weakness, dry mouth, constipation. • May cause impotence.

Nursing Care

■ Abrupt withdrawal may cause life-threatening ↑ BP or dysrhythmias; report to primary health-care provider any dyspnea, severe dizziness, persistent headache, ↑ or ↓ BP, ↑ or ↓ P or irregular pulse rate.

■ Assess BP and pulse for rate, rhythm, and volume before administration and routinely; teach to assess pulse daily and BP twice weekly; hold medication if pulse is below preset parameter such as 50 beats per minute (bpm).

- Assess for ↑ fluid volume: ↑ BP, ↑ intake more than output,↑ weight, edema, breath sounds for crackles, bounding pulse, distended neck veins.
- IV route: Assess VS every 5–15 min, electrocardiogram (ECG), pulmonary capillary wedge pressure.
- Teach to take at same time of day; do not crush, break, or chew extended-release tabs.
- Avoid OTC medications, particularly cold remedies.
- Ensure safety related to orthostatic hypotension, avoidance of hazardous activities.
- Encourage actions to ↓ BP such as ↓ weight, ↓ Na diet, ↑ exercise, ↑ smoking and alcohol intake, stress management.
- Assess for headache, hypotension, dizziness, nausea, dysrhythmias, ↓ sensitivity to cold, impotence.
- *Calcium channel blockers*: Avoid use of calcium-containing antacids or calcium supplements.

Antilipidemics (Lipid Lowering): Decrease Serum LDL, Triglycerides, and Total Cholesterol Levels and Increase HDL Levels

Mechanism of Action	Examples	Nontherapeutic Effects
HMG-CoA reductase inhibitors (statins) Inhibit (HMG-CoA—a catalyst in the synthesis of cholesterol.	atorvastatin (Lipitor) rosuvastatin (Crestor) simvastatin (Zocor)	• N&V, abdominal cramps, diarrhea, constipation, muscle soreness, hepatotoxicity, ↑ absorption of fat-soluble vitamins. *Atorvastatin, rosuvastatin, simvastatin, fenofibrate*: signs of rhabdomyolysis such as arthralgia, arthritis, myalgia, myositis. • *Ezetimibe*: angioedema.
Bile acid sequestrants Bind cholesterol in GI tract.	cholestyramine (Questran)	
Fibrates Inhibit peripheral lipolysis; ↑ triglyceride production and synthesis.	fenofibrate (Tricor) gemfibrozil (Lopid)	

Mechanism of Action	Examples	Nontherapeutic Effects
Cholesterol absorption inhibitors Inhibit absorption of cholesterol in small intestine.	ezetimibe (Zetia)	
Water-soluble vitamins Inhibit release of free fatty acids from adipose tissue; ↓ hepatic lipoprotein synthesis.	niacin	

Nursing Care

- Report occurrence of muscle pain, tenderness, or weakness with fever or malaise; fibrates may ↑ effect of warfarin.
- Encourage ↓ cholesterol, ↓ fat, ↑ fiber; fish high in omega-3 fatty acids 2–3 times a week in diet.
- Monitor serum cholesterol, triglycerides, Hb, red blood cells (RBCs), liver function studies.
- Exchange vegetable oils with polyunsaturated fatty acids (PUFA) to those with monounsaturated fatty acids (MUFA).
- HMG-CoA reductase inhibitors: Take at hr of sleep; avoid grapefruit, which ↑ risk of toxicity.
- Bile acid sequestrants: Take before meals with 8 oz of water; contraindicated for patients with phenylketonuria (PKU).
- Cholesterol absorption inhibitors: Explain to avoid these medications during pregnancy and lactation.
- Water-soluble vitamins: Explain that transient sensation of warmth may occur; ensure safety if orthostatic hypotension occurs.

Antineoplastics and Related Medications: Destroy or Decrease Growth of Neoplastic Cells to Cure, Control, and/or Palliate

Mechanism of Action	Examples	Nontherapeutic Effects
Alkylating agents ↑ DNA synthesis preventing replication.	carboplatin (Paraplatin) cisplatin (Platinol) cyclophosphamide (Cytoxan)	• S&S of myelosuppression such as ↑ white blood cells (WBCs), ↑ platelets. • Skin problems, second malignancies, hypersensitivity, nephrotoxicity, hepatotoxicity, • *Cisplatin:* Ototoxicity, neuropathies, vesicant. • *Cyclophosphamide:* Hemorrhagic cystitis.
Antiandrogens Block testosterone effect at cellular level.	bicalutamide (Casodex) flutamide	Hot flashes, gynecomastia, ↑ libido.
Antiangiogenic agents ↑ new blood vessel formation in tumors.	bevacizumab (Avastin) thalidomide (Thalomid)	• *Bevacizumab:* Hypersensitivity, GI perforation, hypertension, hypertension (HTN), bleeding, ↑ wound healing, arterial thromboembolic events. • *Thalidomide:* Birth defects, sedation, neuropathy, orthostatic hypotension, edema, ↑ WBCs.

Mechanism of Action	Examples	Nontherapeutic Effects
Antiestrogens Compete for estrogen-binding sites in tissue; ↓ aromatase, which ↓ estrogen level.	*Estrogen-binding agents:* tamoxifen citrate *Aromatase inhibitors:* anastrozole (Arimidex) letrozole (Femara)	• *Estrogen-binding agents:* Hot flashes, N&V, ↓ libido, vaginal bleeding. • *Aromatase inhibitors:* Headache, weakness, hot flashes, musculoskeletal pain.
Antimetabolites ↓ DNA synthesis and metabolism; cell-cycle S-phase specific.	capecitabine (Xeloda) fluorouracil or 5-FU (Carac, Efudex, Fluoroplex) gemcitabine (Gemzar) hydroxyurea (Hydrea) methotrexate (Trexall)	Myelosuppression, GI and skin problems, alopecia.
Antitumor antibiotics ↓ DNA synthesis; doxorubicin is cell-cycle S-phase specific.	bleomycin doxorubicin (Doxil) mitomycin	• Myelosuppression, alopecia, skin and GI problems, organ toxicity. • *Bleomycin:* Pulmonary toxicity. • *Doxorubicin:* Red urine, cardiotoxicity.
Cytokines— Hematopoietic growth factors ↑ proliferation and function of hematopoietic cells.	*Increase RBCs:* epoetin alfa (Procrit, Epogen) *Increase WBCs:* filgrastim (Neupogen) pegfilgrastim (Neulasta)	Bone and injection site pain, N&V.
Cytokines— Immune stimulants Suppress cell proliferation.	interferon alpha-2a (Roferon-A) interferon alpha-2b (Intron-A)	Flulike symptoms, myelosuppression.
Monoclonal antibodies Bind to specific receptor sites to ↓ cell proliferation.	cetuximab (Erbitux) rituximab (Rituxan) trastuzumab (Herceptin)	• Fever, N&V, headache, hypersensitivity. • *Cetuximab:* Rash, interstitial lung disease. • *Rituximab:* Tumor lysis syndrome, myelosuppression. • *Trastuzumab:* Diarrhea, cardiotoxicity.

Continued

Mechanism of Action	Examples	Nontherapeutic Effects
Plant alkaloids ↓ cell replication, cell-cycle specific.	docetaxel (Taxotere) paclitaxel topotecan (Hycamtin) vinblastine vincristine	Alopecia, diarrhea, N&V, myelosuppression, hypersensitivity, neurotoxicity, vesicant.
Tyrosine kinase inhibitors (biological response modifiers) ↓ tumor growth; ↑ cell death.	erlotinib (Tarceva)	N&V, photosensitivity, rash.
Combination therapy Concurrent use of multiple meds to destroy rapidly proliferating cells at different stages of replication; lower doses of each med ↓ toxicity and tumor cell resistance.	*CMF:* cyclophosphamide, methotrexate, fluorouracil *CHOP:* cyclophosphamide, doxorubicin, vincristine, prednisone *ABVD:* doxorubicin, bleomycin, vinblastine, dacarbazine	• Myelosuppression, alopecia, skin and GI problems, organ toxicity. • *Bleomycin:* Pulmonary toxicity. • *Doxorubicin:* Red urine, cardiotoxicity.

Nursing Care: See Tab 7, MEDSURG, Nursing Care for Patients With Cancer or Experiencing Nontherapeutic Effect of Antineoplastic Therapies, p. 178.

Antituberculars: Decrease Cough, Sputum, Fever, Night Sweats and Produce Negative Culture for *M. tuberculosis*

Mechanism of Action	Nontherapeutic Effects
Isoniazid (INH) ↓ mycobacterial cell wall synthesis, interferes with metabolism.	Peripheral neuropathy: Numbness, tingling, paresthesia. Hepatotoxicity: Jaundice, N&V, anorexia, amber urine, weakness, fatigue.

Mechanism of Action	Nontherapeutic Effects
Rifampin ↓ mycobacterial RNA synthesis.	• Thrombocytopenia, hepatotoxicity, red/orange urine and other body fluids. • N&V, abdominal pain, flatulence, diarrhea. • Teratogenic; ↓ effectiveness of oral contraceptives.
Ethambutol ↓ mycobacterial RNA synthesis.	• Optic neuritis: ↓ visual acuity, temporary loss of vision, constriction of visual field, red/green color blindness, photophobia, and eye pain. • Rash.
Pyrazinamide (PZA) Causes cellular destruction.	• Hyperuricemia: Pain in great toe and other joints. • Hepatotoxicity, skin rash, anorexia, N&V.
Combination drugs: INH/rifampin (Rifamate); INH/rifampin/PZA (Rifater).	

Nursing Care

- Assess VS, breath sounds, amount and characteristics of sputum.
- Monitor liver and renal labs, CBC, serum uric acid, visual and auditory tests.
- Obtain specimens for mycobacterial tests to detect possible resistance.
- Encourage avoidance of alcohol to ↓ hepatotoxicity.
- *Isoniazid (INH):* Avoid aluminum-containing antacids within 1 hr of INH; give pyridoxine (vitamin B_6) if prescribed to ↓ neuropathy.
- *Rifampin:* Take on empty stomach.
- *Ethambutol:* Take with food; do not breastfeed; eye exams monthly.
- *Pyrazinamide (PZA):* ↑ fluid to 2–3 L daily.

Antiretrovirals Treat HIV and AIDS and Prevent or Decrease Severity of Viral Infections

Mechanism of Action	Examples
Nucleoside reverse transcriptase inhibitors (NRTIs) Damage HIV's DNA interfering with ability to control host DNA.	ABC = abacavir (Ziagen) FTC = emtricitabine (Emtriva) 3TC = lamivudine (Epivir-HBV) ZDV = zidovudine (AZT, Retrovir)

Continued

Mechanism of Action	Examples
Non-nucleoside reverse transcriptase inhibitors (NNRTIs) Prevent conversion of HIV RNA into HIV DNA.	EFV = efavirenz (Sustiva) TDF = tenofovir (Viread)
Protease inhibitors Inhibit HIV protease, preventing virus maturation.	LPV/r = lopinavir/ritonavir (Kaletra) RTV = ritonavir (Norvir)
Multiple drug regimens for naive patients First time on highly active antiretroviral therapy (HAART). EFV + (3TC or FTC) + (ZDV or TDF) LPV/r + (3TC or FTC) + ZDV	Atripla (EFV + TDF + FTC) Combivir (AZT + 3TC) Epzicom (ABC + 3TC) Trizivir (AZT + 3TC + ABC) Truvada (FTC + TDF)

Nontherapeutic Effects

- Anorexia, N&V, diarrhea, headache, dizziness, vaginitis, moniliasis.
- *Additional effects depending on drug:* Confusion, skin eruptions, allergic response, neuropathies, nephrotoxicity, blood dyscrasias, hepatotoxicity, CNS depression.

Nursing Care

- Explain that GI discomfort and insomnia resolve after 3–4 weeks of treatment.
- Refer to manufacturer's insert about need to take with or without food and what to do if a dose is missed.
- Take medications exactly as prescribed; avoid OTC medications; compliance of 95% necessary to prevent resistance.
- Assess for S&S of opportunistic infections, nephrotoxicity, hepatotoxicity, blood dyscrasias.
- Encourage routine medical supervision; blood studies every 2 months.
- Encourage sexual abstinence or use of safer sex practices.

Antivirals Prevent or Decrease Severity of Viral Infections but Do Not Cure

Mechanism of Action	Examples	Nontherapeutic Effects
↓ entry of virus into host to decrease effect of influenza type A.	oseltamivir (Tamiflu)	• Anorexia, N&V, diarrhea, headache, dizziness, vaginitis, moniliasis.
↓ viral DNA synthesis to prevent or limit episodes of herpes simplex, genitalis, zoster, and varicella.	acyclovir (Zovirax) valacyclovir (Valtrex)	• *Depending on med:* Skin eruptions, allergic response, neuropathies, nephrotoxicity, CNS depression, blood dyscrasias, confusion, hepatotoxicity.
↓ viral DNA synthesis to prevent or limit cytomegalovirus, blood dyscrasias.	ganciclovir (Cytovene)	

Nursing Care
- Obtain C&S before starting therapy.
- Take medications exactly as prescribed to maintain blood levels; avoid OTC medications.
- Assess for S&S of nephrotoxicity, hepatotoxicity, blood dyscrasias, opportunistic infections.
- *Oseltamivir:* Begin treatment as soon as S&S appear.
- *Acyclovir, valacyclovir:* Take for pain and pruritus, which usually occur before eruptions; ↑ fluids to 3 L/day; herpes genitalis: ↑ risk for cervical cancer, avoid sexual activity during exacerbations.
- *Ganciclovir:* Give with food; assess for neutropenia, thrombocytopenia, photosensitivity, ↓ visual acuity; ensure regular ophthalmological exams; avoid pregnancy during and for 90 days after treatment (teratogenic); may cause infertility.

Bronchodilators: Promote Bronchial Expansion, Increase Transfer of Gases, Decrease Wheezing and Dyspnea

Mechanism of Action	Examples	Nontherapeutic Effects
Sympathomimetics (beta-adrenergic agonist) Relax bronchial smooth muscle; ↑ spasms.	albuterol (Proventil) metaproterenol terbutaline	Headache, restlessness, tremor, paradoxical bronchospasm evidenced by wheezing, dyspnea, tightness in chest.
Xanthines Relax bronchial smooth muscle; ↑ spasms.	theophylline	↑ P, ↓ BP palpitations, dysrhythmias, nausea, dizziness, headache, restlessness.
Anticholinergics ↑ action of acetylcholine receptor in bronchial smooth muscle.	ipratropium (Atrovent)	Dizziness, headache, nervousness, ↑ BP, palpitations, blurred vision, urinary retention, dry mouth.
Leukotriene receptor antagonists ↓ edema, inflammation.	montelukast (Singulair)	Headache, weakness, N&V.
Inhaled and nasal route steroids ↑ local inflammatory response and edema, ↓ airway diameter.	budesonide (Pulmicort) fluticasone (Flovent)	• Headache, oropharyngeal fungal infections, dysphonia, hoarseness. • Budesonide: Flulike syndrome.

Nursing Care
- Wait 1–5 min between inhaled medications; use bronchodilator first.
- Use spacer with metered dose inhaler (MDI) to limit large droplets; rinse mouth and MDI after use.
- Obtain return demonstration of use of meter, inhaler, nebulizer.
- Assess breath sounds, extent of wheezing, amount and characteristics of sputum.
- Assess respiration (R) rate, depth, characteristics; check heart for ↑ rate and dysrhythmias; ↑ or ↓ BP
- Encourage use of all medications because of variety of purposes.

- Teach to avoid smoking and other respiratory irritants.
- Encourage intake of 2–3 L of fluid daily to help liquefy respiratory secretions.
- Report if shortness of breath (SOB) is not ↓ or is accompanied by diaphoresis, dizziness, palpitations, chest pain.
- *Xanthines*: Use cautiously for patients with cardiac problems because it may ↑ P; give with food; monitor serum theophylline level (therapeutic: 10–20 mcg/mL).
- *Anticholinergics*: Ensure patient does not have glaucoma because it ↑ intraocular pressure; encourage voiding before taking to ↓ urinary retention; suggest lozenges to ↓ dry mouth.
- *Leukotriene receptor antagonists:* Give on empty stomach.
- *Sympathomimetics:* Use cautiously for patients with cardiac problems; avoid use with tricyclic antidepressants or MAO inhibitors because it may cause hypertensive crisis or dysrhythmias.

Antisecretory Agents: Decrease Gastric Acidity and Epigastric Pain

Mechanism of Action	Examples	Nontherapeutic Effects
H_2 antagonists ↓ histamine at H_2 receptors in parietal cells promotes ↓ gastric secretions.	famotidine (Pepcid) ranitidine (Zantac)	• Blood dyscrasias such as ↓ RBCs, ↓ WBCs, ↓ platelets. • CNS disturbances such as confusion, dizziness, drowsiness, headache. • Dysrhythmias, nephrotoxicity, hypersensitivity reactions. • Osteoporosis with long-term use.
Proton pump inhibitors ↓ entry of hydrogen ions into gastric lumen.	esomeprazole (Nexium) lansoprazole (Prevacid) omeprazole (Prilosec) pantoprazole (Protonix)	

Nursing Care

- May ↑ anticoagulant effect of warfarin; CNS disturbances often occur in older adults.
- Give 1–2 hr before or after antacids; give oral medications with meals.
- Assess heart rate and rhythm, emesis and stool for frank or occult blood, CBC for blood dyscrasias.
- *H_2 antagonists:* Teach that smoking interferes with drug action, may cause diarrhea.
- *Proton pump inhibitors:* Advise not to crush or chew capsule.

Diuretics: Increase Urine Output and Decrease Hypervolemia, BP, Peripheral Edema, ICP, Intraocular Pressure, and Seizures

Mechanism of Action	Examples	Nontherapeutic Effects
Thiazides and thiazide-like ↑ sodium (Na) and chloride resorption in distal convoluted tubule and ↑ chloride resorption in ascending loop of Henle.	*Thiazide:* hydrochloroth-iazide (HCTZ) *Thiazide-like:* metolazone (Zaroxolyn)	• Dehydration, orthostatic hypotension, F&E imbalances. • ↑ potassium except with potassium-sparing meds. ↓ potassium with potassium-sparing meds. • ↑ Na, ↓ chloride. • ↑ magnesium, ↓ calcium. • Pain in great toe and other joints.
Loop ↑ Na and chloride resorption in ascending loop of Henle and distal renal tubule	furosemide (Lasix) bumetanide (Bumex)	
Potassium-sparing *Spironolactone:* Acts in distal tubule; ↓ action of aldosterone. ↓ Na, and ↑ potassium excretion. *Triamterene:* ↑ excretion of Na and blocks potassium loss.	spironolactone (Aldactone) triamterene (Dyrenium)	• CNS complications such as dizziness, drowsiness, lethargy, weakness, hearing loss. • N&V, photosensitivity, pulmonary edema, ↓ serum glucose.
Carbonic anhydrase inhibitors diuretic effect ↑ carbonic anhydrase in proximal renal tubule, thereby ↓ excretion of Na, potassium, bicarbonate, and water. *Ophthalmic effect:* ↑ aqueous humor, which ↑ intraocular pressure. *Anticonvulsant effect:* ↑ abnormal paroxysmal discharge in CNS neurons.	acetazolamide (Diamox)	

Nursing Care

- Assess VS before administration; give in a.m. to ↓ disruption in sleep.
- Assess for F&E imbalances, particularly hypo- and hyperkalemia, which can cause dysrhythmias.
- Assess for S&S of hypervolemia such as ↑ BP, bounding pulse, intake exceeds output, ↑ weight, pitting edema, crackles in lungs.
- Assess for S&S of hypovolemia such as ↓ BP, thready pulse, tenting of skin, dry sticky mucous membranes.
- Change position slowly to ↓ orthostatic hypotension.
- Avoid sun to ↓ photosensitivity; suggest use of sunscreen, protective clothing.
- Take medications even if feeling better because medications control, not cure, hypertension.
- Encourage other interventions to ↓ BP such as ↓ weight, low Na diet, ↓ smoking, ↑ exercise and stress management.

Thrombolytic Agents: Dissolve Clots in Blood Vessels or Venous and Arterial Catheters

Mechanism of Action	Examples	Nontherapeutic Effects
Activate conversion of plasminogen to plasmin, which breaks down clots.	alteplase (Activase, t-PA) reteplase (Retavase)	• Bleeding: GI, genitourinary (GU), retroperitoneal, CNS; ecchymoses. • Reperfusion arrhythmias, rash, dyspnea, anaphylaxis.

Nursing Care

- Give within 6 hr of event, preferably 3 hr for a coronary artery thrombi; also given for pulmonary emboli, acute ischemic brain attack, deep vein thrombosis (DVT), arterial thromboembolism, occluded central venous access devices.
- *Identify patients at ↑ risk of bleeding:* >75 yr; ≤10 days postpartum; or receiving warfarin, aspirin, NSAIDs, heparin, heparin-like agents.
- *Identify patients with conditions that contraindicate therapy:* History of brain attack, recent surgery or trauma, uncontrolled HTN, bleeding tendencies, intracranial neoplasm, atriovenous (AV) malformation.
- Follow manufacturer's directions for solution and medication compatibility and infusion rate; use IV infusion pump.
- Assess VS and for bleeding every 15 min 1st hr, every 15–30 min next 8 hr, and then every 4 hr; assess for coffee-ground emesis, tarry stool, occult blood, hematuria, epistaxis; ↓ neurological status, sudden severe

headache, indicating cranial bleeding; joint pain, back and leg pain, indicating retroperitoneal bleeding; abdominal pain, T 104°F, indicating internal bleeding; hold med and call primary health-care provider immediately.
■ Monitor Hb, Hct, platelets, activated partial thromboplastin time (APTT), prothrombin time (PT), thrombin time (TT), INR, and bleeding time.
■ Have blood and antidote aminocaproic acid (Amicar) available to treat hemorrhage.

Hypoglycemics (Oral): Control Blood Glucose in Type 2 Diabetes

Mechanism of Action	Examples	Nontherapeutic Effects
Sulfonylureas Stimulate beta cells to release insulin.	glimepiride (Amaryl) glipizide (Glucotrol) glyburide	Hypoglycemia.
Biguanides ↑ sensitivity to insulin, ↑ binding of insulin to its receptor.	metformin (Glucophage)	• Lactic acidosis: Drowsiness, hyperventilation, myalgia, malaise. • Hypoglycemia.
Meglitinides ↑ release of insulin in pancreas.	repaglinide (Prandin)	Hypoglycemia.
Thiazolidinediones ↑ insulin action in muscle and fat, ↓ gluconeogenesis.	pioglitazone (Actos) rosiglitazone (Avandia)	• Upper respiratory tract infection. • Hypoglycemia does not occur.

Nursing Care

■ *Identify patients with conditions that contraindicate therapy:* Uncontrolled infection; pregnancy; breastfeeding; serious burns; trauma; renal, hepatic, or endocrine disease.
■ Assess for hypoglycemia, hyperglycemia, and hyperosmolar nonketotic coma.
■ Perform finger stick for serum glucose; ketones in urine if blood glucose is ≥300.
■ Teach to avoid alcohol because it may produce Antabuse-like reaction.
■ Teach to not crush sustained-release tablets; take 30 min before meal or follow prescription exactly.
■ *Thiazolidinediones:* Monitor liver function.
■ For hyper- and hypoglycemia and related nursing care, see Tab 6, MEDSURG, Alterations in Blood Glucose Associated With DM, Nursing Care, p. 192.

Insulins: Time-Action Profile of Different Insulins

Insulin Type	Examples	Onset	Peak	Duration
Rapid acting	lispro (Humalog)	15–30 min	30 min–1.5 hr	3–4 hr
	aspart (NovoLog)	10–20 min	1–3 hr	3–5 hr
	glulisine (Apidra)	15–30 min	30 min–1.5 hr	3–4 hr
Short acting	regular (Novolin R)	30–60 min	2–5 hr	5–8 hr
	regular (Humulin R)	30–60 min	1–5 hr	6–10 hr
Intermediate acting	NPH (N) Novolin N Humulin N	1.5–4 hr	4–12 hr	18–24 hr
Long acting	glargine (Lantus)	1–1.5 hr	Steadily delivered, no peak action	20–24 hr
	Detemir (Levemir)	50 min–2 hr	Unknown	24 hr
Premixed	Novolin 70/30	30 min	2–12 hr	24 hr
	Humulin 70/30	30 min	2–4 hr	14–24 hr
	NovoLog Mix 70/30	10–20 min	1–4 hr	24 hr
	Humulin 50/50	30 min	2–5 hr	18–24 hr
	Humalog 75/25	15 min	30 min–2.5 hr	16–20 hr

Nursing Care

- Only regular insulin can be given via IV; rapid-insulin analogs such as aspart and glulisine may be given IV in selective situations with medical supervision.
- Roll, do not shake vials of insulin.
- Use calibrated insulin syringe to ensure accurate dose.

- Give prescribed dose of insulin based on blood glucose levels; usually before meals and before bedtime.

■ Procedure for mixing insulins:

- Proper technique prevents NPH insulin from ↓ purity of solution in the short-acting regular insulin vial.

1. Use insulin syringe calibrated in units (0.3, 0.5, 1 mL; 1/2-, 5/8-, 1-inch needle).
2. Draw up air equal to combined volume of both insulins.
3. Inject NPH vial with amount of air equal to prescribed amount of NPH without dipping needle into solution while keeping vial right-side up.
4. Inject remaining air into regular insulin vial, keep vial right-side up.
5. Invert vial, and draw up the prescribed amount of regular insulin; expel any air or bubbles.
6. Reinsert needle into NPH vial, invert vial, and withdraw prescribed amount.
7. Administer within 5 min of preparation or insulins will bind, decreasing their action.

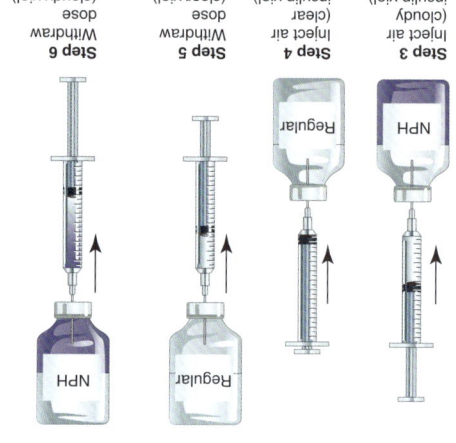

Step 3	**Step 4**	**Step 5**	**Step 6**
Inject air (cloudy insulin vial).	Inject air (clear insulin vial).	Withdraw dose (clear vial).	Withdraw dose (cloudy vial).

Total dose is mixture of clear and cloudy insulins.

Laxatives and Cathartics Decrease Constipation and Promote Evacuation of Bowel

Mechanism of Action	Examples	Nontherapeutic Effects
Bulk-forming laxatives and cathartics ↑ bulk stimulates peristalsis.	methylcellulose (Citrucel) psyllium (Metamucil)	Cramps, F&E imbalances, dependence.
Stool softeners cause water and fat to enter feces to soften and ↓ drying of stool.	docusate sodium (Colace)	
Stimulant and irritants irritate mucosa, causing rapid propulsion of contents.	bisacodyl (Dulcolax) senna (Senokot)	
Lubricants soften feces.	Mineral oil	
Saline osmotics draw water into intestinal lumen, distending bowel and stimulating peristalsis.	magnesium salts (Milk of Magnesia) sodium phosphate (Fleet Phospho-Soda)	

Nursing Care

- Identify patients for whom the medication is contraindicated: N&V, abdominal pain, or S&S of acute abdomen because these may indicate bowel obstruction; do not use sodium osmotic with older adults or children because it may cause F&E imbalances.
- Give at bedtime.
- Encourage ↑ fluid intake, activity, dietary fiber; assess stool frequency, consistency.
- *Bulk-forming:* Teach to mix in 8 oz of fluid and follow with 8 oz fluid; may take ≥12 hr to act.
- *Stool softeners:* Inform that results may take several days to act.
- *Stimulants/irritants:* Inform that results occur quickly; fluid may be passed with feces.
- *Lubricants:* Inform that absorption of fat-soluble vitamins may decrease.
- *Saline osmotics:* Inform that results occur quickly; monitor for S&S of dehydration, hypernatremia, ↓ absorption of fat-soluble vitamins.

Opioid (Narcotic) Antagonists: Reverse Opioid-Induced CNS Depression and Decreased Respiratory Function

Mechanism of Action	Examples	Nontherapeutic Effects
Displace opioid at receptor sites via competitive antagonism.	naltrexone	N&V, abdominal cramps, muscle and joint pain, insomnia, anxiety, headache, hepatotoxicity; may cause early fetal loss.
	naloxone	N&V, ↓ or ↑ BP, ventricular fibrillation.

Nursing Care

■ Assess VS, particularly respiratory rate and BP.
■ Assess for S&S of opioid withdrawal such as restlessness, ↑ BP, ↑ temp, abdominal cramps, and N&V.

Opioid (Narcotic) Analgesics Decrease Transmission of Pain Impulses, Coughing, and GI Motility

Mechanism of Action	Examples	Nontherapeutic Effects
Combine with opioid receptors in CNS.	codeine fentanyl (Duragesic): 72-hr transdermal patch hydrocodone (Hycodan) hydromorphone (Dilaudid) methadone (Dolophine) morphine (MS Contin) oxycodone (OxyContin)	• ↓ R, sedation, constipation, nausea, drowsiness, pruritus. • *Fentanyl:* Dry mouth, diaphoresis, weakness.

Opioid and Nonopioid Analgesic Combinations Provide More Effective Pain Relief Due to Synergistic Effect

- Codeine phosphate and acetaminophen (Tylenol with codeine 1, 2, 3, or 4).
- Hydrocodone and acetaminophen (Vicodin).
- Oxycodone and acetaminophen (Percocet).
- Oxycodone and aspirin (Percodan).

Nursing Care

- Assess for respiratory depression; if respiratory rate is ≤10 breaths per min, hold dose and call primary health-care provider.
- Keep opioid antagonist available, such as naloxone, naltrexone, for toxicity or overdose.
- Assess pain, VS, ↓ BP, drowsiness, confusion, constipation, N&V, tolerance and dependence.
- Give before pain is severe because regularly scheduled doses maintain therapeutic blood levels and ↑ effectiveness.
- Give additional prescribed medication for breakthrough pain; common with continuous infusion, sustained-release medication, or intractable pain.
- Give cautiously because combinations ↑ effectiveness (synergistic effect) and may ↑ risk of toxicity.
- Decrease slowly after chronic use to ↓ S&S of withdrawal.
- Encourage coughing and deep breathing every 2 hr.
- Increase fluids, fiber, and activity to limit constipation; give prescribed stool softeners and laxatives.
- Provide for safety; encourage avoidance of hazardous activities; change position slowly.
- Use cautiously with ↑ intracranial pressure (ICP) because it can mask S&S of increasing ICP.
- Teach how to self-administer medications such as intramuscular (IM), subcutaneous (sub-Q), sublingual, transdermal.

Antiseizure Agents Decrease Occurrence, Frequency, and/or Severity of Seizures

Mechanism of Action	Examples	Nontherapeutic Effects
Action depends on drug classification.	acetazolamide (Diamox)	• Drowsiness, dizziness, N&V, rash, headache.
Seizure Type:	carbamazepine (Tegretol)	• ↓ BP, respiratory depression.
Focal	gabapentin (Neurontin)	• Blood dyscrasias such as ↑ WBCs, ↑ RBCs, ↑ platelets.
Generalized	lamotrigine (Lamictal)	• Hepatotoxicity.
Tonic-clonic	levetiracetam (Keppra)	
Absence	topiramate (Topamax)	
Myoclonic	valproates (Depakote, Depakene)	
Tonic	*Status epilepticus:*	
Atonic	diazepam (Valium)	
Clonic	lorazepam (Ativan)	
Status epilepticus (acute prolonged seizure activity)		

Nursing Care

- Increase gradually as prescribed until seizure control is achieved; may require two antiseizure medications.
- Shake suspensions before administration; give with food to ↓ GI irritation.
- Monitor serum drug levels (e.g., phenytoin: therapeutic 10–20 mcg/L, toxic 30–50 mcg/L).
- Teach that medication may be continued indefinitely; withdrawal may be attempted after 3 yr of being seizure-free.
- Advise that there may be some ↓ effectiveness of oral contraceptives; advise to consult primary health-care provider when planning pregnancy or lactation.
- **Withdraw medication over 6–12 weeks because seizures occur with abrupt withdrawal.**
- Status epilepticus: Give prescribed IV diazepam (Valium) or lorazepam (Ativan); keep resuscitative equipment available.

Bone Resorption Inhibitors: Decrease Bone Resorption and Potential for Fractures and Increase Bone Density

Mechanism of Action	Examples	Nontherapeutic Effects

Bisphosphonates
↓ osteoclast activity,
↓ bone resorption.
	alendronate (Fosamax)
	ibandronate (Boniva)
	pamidronate (Aredia)
	risedronate (Actonel)
	zoledronic acid (Reclast,
	Zometa)
		• N&V, diarrhea,
		  bone pain, abdom-
		  inal pain, flushing.
		• May cause
		  osteonecrosis of
		  jaw.

Hormonal agents
Opposes effects of
parathyroid hormone.
	calcitonin salmon
	(Miacalcin)
	teriparatide (Forteo)
		• Transient N&V,
		  diarrhea.
		• Flushing and/or
		  warmth 1 hr after
		  IM or sub-Q
		• *Calcitonin salmon:*
		  Nasal irritation
		  with nasal route.

Nursing Care

- Teach effect takes >1 month.
- Assess for hypocalcemia such as ↓ BP, muscle spasms, paresthesias, laryngospasm, positive Chvostek and/or Trousseau signs.
- Teach to discuss plans for pregnancy or lactation with primary health-care provider.
- Encourage intake of calcium foods and prescribed calcium and vitamin D supplements.
- Encourage weight-bearing exercise; avoid smoking, alcohol, and cola, which ↑ osteoporosis; ensure baseline bone density test.
- *Bisphosphonates:* Teach to take oral dose in a.m. with water on empty stomach.
- *Calcitonin salmon:* Perform intradermal allergy test first because medication may cause anaphylaxis; alternate nostrils daily with intranasal calcitonin.

Obstetric Medications

Uterine relaxants: Magnesium sulfate, terbutaline, indomethacin (Indocin)
- *Action:* ↓ uterine contractions.
- *Contraindications:* HTN, DM, preeclampsia, <20 or >36 weeks' gestation.
- *Nursing care:* Use infusion pump; assess VS, BP, S&S of preterm labor, tremor, absence of deep tendon reflexes; provide emotional support; hold magnesium if knee-jerk reflex absent.

Uterine stimulants for labor: Oxytocin (Pitocin), misoprostol (Cytotec)
- *Action:* ↑ uterine contractions.
- *Contraindications:* Cephalopelvic disproportion, malpresentation, nonreassuring fetal signs, placenta previa, active genital herpes, uterine scar.
- *Nursing care:* Assess fetal heart rate and S&S of shock; discontinue if contractions are less than 2-min intervals or last more than 90 seconds, then use left side-lying position, oxygen; prepare for cesarean birth.

Uterine stimulants to decrease postpartum bleeding: Carboprost (Hemabate), methylergonovine (Methergine), ergonovine (Ergotrate)
- *Action:* ↑ uterine tone to treat postpartum bleeding.
- *Nursing care:* Assess for bleeding and N&V; Give antidiarrheal if prescribed.

Uterine evacuation: Misoprostol (Cytotec), dinoprostone (Cervidil)
- *Action:* Elective abortion 12–28 weeks' gestation, after missed abortion or fetal demise.
- *Nursing care:* Insert following manufacturer's directions; assess progress; dinoprostone: Assess for ↑ temp; notify primary health-care provider of chest tightness.

Cervical softening agents: Dinoprostone (Prostin E2, Cervidil)
- *Action:* Cervical softening agents ↑ effacement; followed by oxytocin to stimulate contractions.
- *Nursing care:* Insert gel or suppository following manufacturer's directions; assess fetal status, progress of labor; dinoprostone: Assess for ↑ temp; notify primary health-care provider of chest tightness due to ↑ sensitivity.

Immune globulins: Rh₀(D) immune globulin (RhoGAM) immune globulin microdose
- *Action:* Prevent isoimmunization in Rh-negative patient exposed to Rh-positive RBCs; protect against erythroblastosis fetalis in next Rh-positive pregnancy.

- *Nursing care:* Give within 72 hr after birth or termination to eligible mother only; ensure vial is cross-matched to woman.

Anticonvulsant: Magnesium sulfate

- *Action:* ↓ seizures in preeclampsia.
- *Nursing care:* Assess for ↓ BP, ↓ R, pulse for rate and rhythm; seizure precautions; magnesium sulfate: Assess pulmonary and neurological status; discontinue for tightness in chest or absence of knee-jerk reflex; serum magnesium levels every 6 hr; warm flush is expected.

Antihypertensives: Hydralazine, labetalol, nifedipine (Procardia)

- *Action:* ↓ BP in preeclampsia.
- *Nursing care:* Assess for ↓ BP, ↑ P, F&E imbalance; maintain supine position during and 3 hr after; assess newborn for hypotension, respiratory depression, hyporeflexia.

Glucocorticoids: Betamethasone (Celestone), dexamethasone

- *Action:* ↓ neonatal respiratory distress syndrome.
- *Nursing care:* Assess for F&E imbalance, cerebral edema; S&S of adrenal insufficiency such as ↑ weight, ↑ BP, weakness, N&V, lethargy, confusion, restlessness; discontinue slowly if used more than 1 week.

Skeletal muscle relaxants: Central acting—cyclobenzaprine (Flexeril), diazepam (Valium); direct acting—dantrolene (Dantrium)

- *Action:* ↓ muscle spasms.
  - Central acting: Interfere with reflexes in upper CNS.
  - Direct acting: Interfere with release of calcium from muscle tubules within skeletal muscles, preventing contraction.
- *Nursing care:* Give with food or milk to ↓ GI irritation; avoid hazardous activity until sedative effect is known; avoid alcohol and other CNS depressants; ↓ constipation by ↑ fluids, ↑ fiber, prescribed stool softeners; assess pain, muscle stiffness, ROM routinely; encourage rest and ordered heat, physical therapy.

Hormonal Disorders and Related Medications

- Do not discontinue any hormonal medications abruptly.

Hyperthyroidism

- **Propylthiouracil (PTU), methimazole (Tapazole)**
  - *Action:* ↓ formation of thyroid hormone.
  - *Nontherapeutic effects:* Agranulocytosis evidenced by sore throat, fever, headache, malaise.

- *Nursing care:* Report S&S of agranulocytosis to primary health-care provider.
- **Radioactive iodine:** ^{131}I (atomic cocktail)
  - *Action:* Destroy thyroid tissue.
  - *Nontherapeutic effects:* S&S of hypothyroidism such as fatigue, lethargy, ↓ weight, cold intolerance, constipation, dry skin.
  - *Nursing care:* Use precautions for 6–8 hr to 3–7 days as ordered, such as discard vomitus and excreta with multiple toilet flushes, avoid holding or hugging others, isolation from others.

Hypothyroidism

- **Levothyroxine sodium (Synthroid, Levothyroid)**
  - *Action:* Replace thyroid hormone.
  - *Nontherapeutic effects:* S&S of hyperthyroidism such as ↑ VS, irritability, insomnia, headache, dysrhythmias, ↑ weight, diaphoresis, diarrhea, heat intolerance, fine hand tremor.
  - *Nursing care:* Hold medication and notify primary health-care provider for resting pulse ≥100 per min.

Hyperparathyroidism

- **Calcitonin (Miacalcin)**
  - *Action:* ↑ renal excretion of calcium.
  - *Nontherapeutic effects:* Facial flushing, injection site reactions, hypersensitivity, hypocalcemia.
  - *Nursing care:* Assess for S&S of hypocalcemia such as muscle twitching, irritability, paresthesias, positive Chvostek and/or Trousseau signs.

Diabetes Insipidus

- **Desmopressin (DDAVP)**
  - *Action:* ↑ water reabsorption by distal renal tubules.
  - *Nontherapeutic effects:* S&S of water intoxication such as confusion, drowsiness, headache, ↑ weight, dysuria, seizures.
  - *Nursing care:* Assess for S&S of water intoxication and dehydration; daily weight, intake and output (I&O).

Cushing Syndrome

- **Mitotane (Lysodren), ketoconazole (Nizoral)**
  - *Action:* ↑ production of adrenal steroids.
  - *Nontherapeutic effects:* N&V, GI distress, depression, rash, vertigo, diplopia, many drug interactions, may precipitate adrenal insufficiency.

- *Nursing care:* Assess VS; S&S for adrenal insufficiency such as fatigue, orthostatic hypotension, ↓ weight, dehydration, GI distress, shock. Mitotane: Assess for ↓ hepatic function.

Addison Disease

- **Hydrocortisone (Cortef)**
  - *Action:* Glucocorticoid and mineralocorticoid replacement therapy.
  - *Nontherapeutic effects:* Na and fluid retention;↓ wound healing; anaphylaxis; ↑ weight; urinary frequency, urgency; vertigo; thrombophlebitis; and other CNS and cardiovascular problems.
  - *Nursing care:* Generally larger dose in a.m. than afternoon as prescribed because it mimics circadian rhythm and decreases side effects; ↑ dose when stressed; assess VS, daily weight, F&E balance; protect from infection because medication masks infection; minimize noise, light, extremes in environmental temperature.
- **Fludrocortisone**
  - *Action:* Mineralocorticoid replacement to manage Na loss and ↓ BP.
  - *Nontherapeutic effects:* Heart failure, dizziness, headache, hypokalemia, adrenal suppression, ↑ weight, edema.
  - *Nursing care:* Assess VS, fluid retention, electrolyte imbalances; ↓ BP may indicate inadequate dose.

Hyperpituitarism

- **Octreotide (Sandostatin)**
  - *Action:* ↓ growth hormone levels.
  - *Nontherapeutic effects:* Dizziness, drowsiness, orthostatic hypotension, visual disturbances, diarrhea.
  - *Nursing care:* Assess VS, BP, S&S of gallbladder disease, diarrhea; store in refrigerator; give at room temperature.

Premature Menopause and Menopausal Symptoms

- **Estrogen, conjugated (Premarin)**
  - *Action:* Hormone replacement therapy (HRT); used based on risk versus benefit.
  - *Nontherapeutic effects:* Nausea, fluid retention, headache, breast tenderness, oily skin, amenorrhea, dysmenorrhea; contraindicated in pregnancy and breast cancer.
  - *Nursing care:* Assess daily weight and BP for increases due to Na and water retention; assess for and teach S&S of thromboembolic disorders

such as thrombophlebitis (extremity pain, swelling, tenderness), brain attack (headache, blurred vision), pulmonary embolus (chest pain, dyspnea, cough).

Erectile Dysfunction

- **Sildenafil (Viagra), tadalafil (Cialis), alprostadil (Muse)**
  - *Action:* ↑ strength and duration of erections.
  - *Nontherapeutic effects*: HTN, urinary tract infection (UTI), headache, insomnia, constipation, dry mouth, erection lasting ≥4 hr.
  - *Nursing care:* Teach to take 1 hr before intercourse, use only once daily; assess for S&S of cardiac distress, drug interactions; call primary health-care provider if erection lasts ≥4 hr; avoid concurrent use with a nitrate because of risk of fatal brain attack, MI.

Contraception

- **Oral monophasic, biphasic, triphasic formulations (combined estrogen and progestin in different doses and cycles)**
  - *Action:* ↓ ovulation by suppressing follicle-stimulating hormone (FSH) and luteinizing hormone (LH).
  - *Contraindications:* ≥35-yr-old smoker, history of thromboembolism.
  - *Nontherapeutic effects:* Nausea, breakthrough bleeding, vaginal candidiasis, ↑ BP, fluid retention, pigmentation of face, thromboembolism.
  - *Nursing care:* Teach ↑ pregnancy risk with concurrent use of antibiotics, phenobarbital, phenytoin, and rifampin; follow instructions for pill sequence and missed pills; assess for S&S of ectopic pregnancy; avoid breastfeeding; advise to have regular Pap smears, physicals, mammograms; stop smoking.
- **Medroxyprogesterone (Depo-Provera); etonogestrel implant (Implanon)**
  - *Action:* ↓ sperm and ovum transport, ↓ ovum implantation.
  - *Contraindications:* ≥35-yr-old smoker, history of thromboembolism.
  - *Nontherapeutic effects:* Uterine bleeding, thromboembolism. Etonogestrel implant: ↑ BP, headache.
  - *Nursing care:* Teach ↑ pregnancy risk with concurrent use of antibiotics, phenobarbital, phenytoin, rifampin; advise to have regular Pap smears, physicals, mammograms, stop smoking. Medroxyprogesterone: Administer injection 4x/yr. Etonogestrel implant: Assess implant site usually at midportion of upper arm; teach to replace within 3 yr, as effectiveness decreases.

- **Levonorgestrel/ethinylestradiol, levonorgestrel**
  - *Action:* ↓ implantation; 75% effective.
  - *Contraindications:* ≥35-yr-old smoker, history of thromboembolism.
  - *Nontherapeutic effects:* Thromboembolism, nausea, abdominal pain, fatigue, headache, menstrual changes.
  - *Nursing care:* Teach ↑ pregnancy risk with use of antibiotics, phenobarbital, phenytoin, and rifampin; begin within 72 hr after intercourse; refer to contraception counseling.

Prostate Cancer

- **Leuprolide (Lupron Depot, Eligard), goserelin (Zoladex)**
  - *Action:* Produces chemical castration; ↓ testosterone.
  - *Nontherapeutic effects:* Bone pain, hot flashes, ↓ libido, impotence.
  - *Nursing care:* Teach that bone pain resolves with time; give analgesics for pain.
- **Flutamide, bicalutamide (Casodex)**
  - *Action:* Inhibits androgen uptake or binding.
  - *Nontherapeutic effects:* Hot flashes, ↓ libido, impotence, breast pain and gynecomastia, diarrhea, hepatotoxicity.
  - *Nursing care:* Notify primary health-care provider if hepatotoxicity occurs.

Medications for Degenerative Diseases of the Nervous System

Parkinson Disease: Restore Dopamine and Acetylcholine Balance; Decrease Motor S&S Such as Stooped Posture, Nonintention Tremors, Rigidity, Impaired Coordination

Mechanism of Action	Examples	Nontherapeutic Effects
Dopaminergics ↑ dopamine in corpus striatum.	amantadine bromocriptine (Parlodel) carbidopa-levodopa (Sinemet)	• ↓ BP, ↑ P, fatigue, anorexia, N&V, dry mouth, tremors, constipation. • *Toxicity:* Muscle twitching, mood changes. • *Carbidopa-levodopa:* Urine and sweat may darken in color.

Continued

Mechanism of Action	Examples	Nontherapeutic Effects
Anticholinergics ↓ excess cholinergic activity in brain.	benztropine (Cogentin)	Dry mouth, blurred vision, ↑ P, constipation, urinary retention.
COMT inhibitor Inhibits the enzyme COMT, prevents levodopa breakdown.	entacapone (Comtan) tolcapone (Tasmar)	Brownish/orange urine, dyskinesia, N&V, ↓ BP. *Entacapone:* Disintegration of muscle (**rhabdomyolysis**), neuroleptic malignant syndrome.
Monoamine oxidase B inhibitor Inactivates MAO thereby ↑ dopamine.	selegiline (Eldepryl)	CNS stimulation or depression, confusion, dizziness, nausea.

Nursing Care

- Teach effect may take several months; therapy is palliative.
- Give exactly as prescribed and slowly because of dysphagia.
- Encourage eating after taking to use advantage of ↓ dysphagia and to ↓ GI irritation.
- Assess VS; change position slowly; avoid hazardous activity.
- Do not discontinue abruptly because parkinsonian crisis may occur.
- *Dopaminergics:* Teach to avoid food such as veal, lamb, pork, egg yolks, and potatoes that are high in pyridoxine (B_6) because they ↓ effectiveness.
- *Sinemet:* Ensure not given with narrow-angle glaucoma and MAO inhibitors.
- *Anticholinergics:* Provide frequent oral care; encourage use of gum or hard candy to ↑ salivation; give prescribed stool softeners; catheterize for urinary retention if ordered.
- *MAO inhibitors:* Avoid concurrent use with an opioid, SSRI, or tricyclic because it may cause a fatal interaction.

Alzheimer Disease Slows Progressive Deterioration of Cognition and Behavior

Mechanism of Action	Examples	Nontherapeutic Effects
Acetylcholinesterase (AchE) inhibitors ↑ acetylcholine levels in cerebral cortex.	donepezil (Aricept) galantamine (Razadyne) rivastigmine (Exelon)	• Anorexia, N&V, diarrhea, ↓ BP, headache, dizziness, insomnia. • *Overdose:* Severe N&V, diaphoresis, salivation, ↓ P, seizures, ↑ muscle weakness, including respiratory muscles.
N-methyl D-aspartate receptor (NMDAR) antagonist ↓ action of NMDAR.	memantine (Namenda)	Dizziness, confusion, headache, vomiting, constipation.

Nursing Care
- Use with caution in patients with COPD or asthma.
- Teach therapy is palliative and lifelong, not a cure.
- Ensure medication is prescribed in form patient can swallow.
- Monitor VS, respiratory status, Hb, Hct, stool for melena, weekly weight.
- Protect from injury.

Myasthenia Gravis Medications Increase Strength of Skeletal Muscle Contractions

Mechanism of Action	Examples	Nontherapeutic Effects
Anticholinesterase muscle stimulants ↓ cholinesterase, thus ↑ acetylcholine.	ambenonium (Mytelase) edrophonium (Enlon, Tensilon) pyridostigmine (Mestinon)	*Cholinergic S&S:* ↑ salivation, ↑ lacrimation, N&V, diarrhea, intestinal cramping, ↓ P, papillary constriction.

Medications for Cardiac Problems

Antidysrhythmics Decrease Abnormal Electrical Conduction Through Heart

Mechanism of Action	Examples	Nontherapeutic Effects
Class I—calcium ion antagonists Slows conduction; local anesthetic; used for ventricular dysrhythmias.	flecainide (Tambocor) lidocaine procainamide	Heart failure, new dysrhythmias, ↓ BP, GI distress, blood dyscrasias, anticholinergic effects, diarrhea, neurotoxicity.
Class II—β-adrenergic blocker ↓ cardiac excitability, cardiac output, and workload; ↑ heart rate and ↓ BP; used for angina, HTN, and dysrhythmias.	atenolol (Tenormin) metoprolol (Lopressor) nadolol (Corgard) propranolol (Inderal)	
Class III—potassium channel blockers Slows heart rate and conduction; used for ventricular and supraventricular dysrhythmias.	amiodarone (Cordarone) dofetilide (Tikosyn) ibutilide (Corvert)	

Nursing Care

- ■ **Assess for myasthenic crisis:** Dyspnea, dysarthria, respiratory arrest.
- ■ **Assess for cholinergic crisis:** Due to overdose of anticholinergics; ptosis; weakness; difficulty chewing, swallowing, breathing; keep IV atropine sulfate available as antidote for anticholinesterase muscle stimulants.
- ■ Administer edrophonium as prescribed to distinguish between myasthenic crisis (S&S will ↑) from cholinergic crisis (S&S will ↓).
- ■ Give carefully due to dysphagia; give with food or milk to ↓ GI irritation.
- ■ Give medications exactly as scheduled; usually before meals to ↑ chewing and swallowing.
- ■ Have tracheostomy set and resuscitative equipment available.
- ■ Evaluate response as dosage is adjusted accordingly.
- ■ Balance activity and rest; plan activities when strength is greatest.

Mechanism of Action	Examples	Nontherapeutic Effects
Class IV—calcium channel blocker ↓ entry of calcium into myocardial and vascular smooth muscle cells; ↓ SA and AV node conduction; used for atrial fibrillation and supraventricular tachycardia.	diltiazem (Cardizem) felodipine (Plendil) nifedipine (Procardia) verapamil (Calan)	

Nursing Care

- Keep resuscitation equipment available.
- Use infusion controller for IV; assess VS, BP, and ECG continually until stable.
- Obtain heart rate before administration; withhold medication based on preset parameters.
- Monitor therapeutic blood levels.
- Assess for S&S of ↑ fluid volume such as crackles, edema, weight gain.
- Maintain safety; change position slowly to ↓ risk of hypotension.
- Teach about medication regimen; need to ↓ Na intake; report side effects; identify irregular beats or ↑ or ↓ heart rate; need for continued medical supervision.

Cardiac Glycoside: Increases Force of Cardiac Contraction and Cardiac Output and Decreases Heart Rate

Mechanism of Action	Examples	Nontherapeutic Effects
Cardiac glycoside ↑ force of cardiac contraction (positive inotropic effect). ↓ rate of cardiac contractions (negative chronotropic effect). ↓ conduction velocity (negative dromotropic effect).	digoxin (Lanoxin)	• ↓ P, headache, drowsiness, fatigue, weakness. • *Toxicity:* N&V; anorexia; visual disturbances such as blurred, yellow vision; premature ventricular complexes; diarrhea.

Nursing Care

- Initiate digoxin therapy as prescribed (digitalization):
- *Slow method:* Dose gradually increased; used in less acute situations in ambulatory setting.
- *Fast method:* Dose rapidly increased; used in acute heart failure (HF) in hospital setting.
- Teach to take own pulse; hold medication and notify primary health-care provider if less than preset parameters such as <50–60 bpm.
- Teach to recognize S&S of toxicity; call primary health-care provider if they occur.
- Monitor therapeutic blood level (0.8–2 ng/mL); has narrow therapeutic window.
- Monitor potassium levels; notify primary health-care provider if below 3.5 mEq/L because it may precipitate digoxin toxicity.
- Assess for hyperkalemia if on potassium-sparing diuretic.
- Encourage foods high in potassium unless taking potassium-sparing medication.

Cardiac Stimulants: Increase Heart Rate

Mechanism of Action	Examples	Nontherapeutic Effects
Cardiac stimulants Stimulate alpha and beta receptors in the heart to ↑ heart rate, contractility.	atropine sulfate dobutamine epinephrine norepinephrine (Levophed)	• Dysrhythmias, ↑ P, headache, angina. • *Atropine sulfate:* Anticholinergic effects such as dry mouth, blurred vision, urinary retention.

Nursing Care

- Assess VS frequently during administration.
- Monitor ECG continuously when given IV.
- Ensure ongoing follow-up care and ECGs.

Coronary Vasodilators: Dilate Arteries and Decrease Preload, Afterload, and Myocardial Oxygen Consumption

Mechanism of Action	Examples	Nontherapeutic Effects
Coronary vasodilators Mechanism varies by med; blocks calcium channels or relaxes smooth muscle to treat angina, mild hypertension.	amlodipine (Norvasc) isosorbide dinitrate (Isordil, Sorbitrate) nifedipine (Procardia) nitroglycerine (Nitro-Dur, Sublingual Nitrostat) verapamil (Calan)	Orthostatic hypotension, ↑ P, headache, dizziness, N&V, flushing, confusion.

Nursing Care

- Assess BP; hold at set parameters.
- Teach to take prescribed acetaminophen for headache.
- *Nitroglycerine (transdermal):* See Medication Administration, p. 292.
- *Nitroglycerine (sublingual):*
  - Teach to take sip of water; put sublingual tablet under tongue; expect slight tingling as tablet dissolves.
  - Take 1 pill every 5 min up to 3 times for chest pain; if pain continues, get emergency help such as dial 911.
  - Store tablets in dark, tightly closed bottle; medications expire in 6 months.

Psychotropic Medications

Anxiolytics, Sedatives, and Hypnotics Decrease Anxiety, Induce Sleep, Ease Alcohol Withdrawal

Mechanism of Action	Examples	Nontherapeutic Effects
Benzodiazepines ↓ action of gamma-aminobutyric acid (GABA) inhibitory neurotransmitter.	**Short acting** alprazolam (Xanax) midazolam **Medium acting** lorazepam (Ativan) **Long acting** chlordiazepoxide (Librium) clonazepam (Klonopin) diazepam (Valium) buspirone (BuSpar)	↑ mental alertness, ↑ BP, drowsiness, dizziness, headache. • Paradoxical reactions such as euphoria, excitement.
Nonbarbiturates All have CNS-depressant effect, variable action, depending on med.	diphenhydramine (Benadryl) hydroxyzine (Vistaril) zolpidem (Ambien)	

Nursing Care

- Avoid alcohol, as it ↑ effects; avoid caffeine, as it ↑ effects.
- Avoid hazardous activities until tolerance develops.
- Avoid concurrent use with herbal products such as St. John's wort, kava, ginseng.
- Hold medication if systolic BP falls <20 mm Hg on standing.
- Discontinue gradually to prevent S&S of withdrawal; use more than 2 weeks may cause dependence.
- *Buspirone:* Effect takes 3–6 weeks, which is longer than other anxiolytics.

Antidepressants: Lift Depressed Mood, Minimize Panic Response, Narcolepsy, and Attention Deficit Behaviors

Mechanism of Action	Examples	Nontherapeutic Effects
Tricyclics (TCAs) ↓ reuptake of norepinephrine and serotonin into presynaptic nerve terminals.	doxepin (Silenor) imipramine (Tofranil) nortriptyline (Pamelor)	Anticholinergic effects, ↓ BP, CNS stimulation effects.
Selective serotonin reuptake inhibitors (SSRIs) ↓ reuptake of serotonin into presynaptic nerve terminals.	citalopram (Celexa) fluoxetine (Prozac) paroxetine (Paxil) sertraline (Zoloft)	• Sexual dysfunction. • ↑ appetite. • Anticholinergic and CNS stimulation or depression. • Hepatotoxicity, weight gain, photosensitivity.
Monoamine oxidase inhibitors (MAOIs) ↓ breakdown of dopamine, norepinephrine, and serotonin in CNS neurons.	phenelzine (Nardil) selegiline (Eldepryl) tranylcypromine (Parnate)	• Sexual dysfunction, rash, anticholinergic effects. • CNS stimulation or depression.
Atypical new generation medications ↑ effects of dopamine serotonin and/or norepinephrine at neural membranes.	bupropion (Wellbutrin) mirtazapine (Remeron) venlafaxine (Effexor)	Drowsiness, dizziness, headache, insomnia, N&V, anticholinergic effects.

Nursing Care
■ Assess for suicidal potential; especially as mood lifts and physical and psychic energy increase.
■ Ensure minimum of 2–6 weeks between concurrent use of TCAs, MAOIs, or SSRIs to avoid serotonin syndrome; do not discontinue medication abruptly.
■ Assess for anticholinergic and CNS effects.
■ Avoid prescription, OTC, or herbal products without supervision.
■ Take at hr of sleep if sedation occurs or in a.m. if insomnia occurs.
■ Avoid hazardous activities until sedative effect is known.
■ Change positions slowly to ↓ orthostatic hypotension.

Tricyclics
- Avoid giving with narrow-angle glaucoma or cardiac condition.
- Teach effect may take 2–6 weeks.

SSRIs
- Teach effect may take 5 weeks.
- Obtain baseline weight, assess regularly.
- Teach to ↑ exercise and ↓ caloric intake to ↓ weight gain.
- Teach to wear protective clothing and sunscreen outdoors.

MAOIs
- Prevent hypertensive crisis by eliminating foods containing tyramine such as aged cheese, beer, wine, chocolate, caffeine, licorice, bananas, raisins, pepperoni, salami, bologna, liver, sour cream, yogurt.
- Assess BP when given with antihypertensive because hypotension may occur.
- Teach effect may take 4–8 weeks.

New Generation Medications
- Give with food to ↓ GI irritation; teach to not chew or crush sustained-release capsules.
- Teach to avoid alcohol during therapy because of potentiation.
- Assess VS routinely for ↑ BP and ↑ P; ↑ or ↓ weight.
- Institute seizure precautions; assess for S&S of seizure.
- Teach pregnancy classification of medication; notify primary health-care provider if pregnancy is planned.

Antipsychotic Agents Decrease Agitated Behavior, Disorganized Thinking, and Positive and Negative Psychotic Signs and Symptoms

Mechanism of Action	Examples	Nontherapeutic Effects
Typical antipsychotics Specific action depends on med. *↓ positive symptoms:* Delusions, hallucinations, agitation, catatonia, disorganized speech and behavior.	chlorpromazine haloperidol (Haldol) prochlorperazine	• Sedation, ↓ BP, anorexia, sexual dysfunction, anticholinergic effects, photosensitivity; signs of cardiotoxicity, hepatotoxicity, agranulocytosis.

Mechanism of Action	Examples	Nontherapeutic Effects
Atypical antipsychotics Specific action depends on med. ↓ *negative symptoms:* Blunt affect, passivity, apathy, withdrawal, lack of pleasure, inability to decide and speak.	aripiprazole (Abilify) clozapine (Clozaril) olanzapine (Zyprexa) quetiapine (Seroquel) risperidone (Risperdal) ziprasidone (Geodon)	• *Extrapyramidal tract side effects (EPS):* Dystonia (early in therapy); akathisia (most common); parkinsonism, tardive dyskinesia (prolonged use); may be reversible if dose is ↓ or withdrawn but some may be permanent. • *Neuroleptic malignant syndrome:* ↑ temp (cardinal sign), muscular rigidity, tremors, impaired ventilation, unstable BP, autonomic hyperactivity, muteness, altered LOC.

Nursing Care

- Teach effect may take 1–2 weeks; sedation may occur immediately; avoid hazardous activities; avoid coffee, tea, cola, antacids that ↓ medication effectiveness.
- Obtain BP before each dose; hold medication based on systolic and diastolic parameters.
- Assess for ↓ anticholinergic effects; ↑ fluids, ↑ fiber diet, suggest use of hard candy.
- Monitor CBC and liver function studies routinely.
- Assess weight to evaluate response to anorexia and energy expenditure related to extrapyramidal side effects.
- Assess for S&S of cardiotoxicity, particularly during initiation of therapy.
- Teach to limit exposure to sun; wear protective clothing, sunblock, sun glasses.
- Give prescribed medication to ↓ extrapyramidal side effects: benztropine (Cogentin), biperiden (Akineton), clonazepam (Klonopin).
- Give prescribed medications to ↓ neuroleptic malignant syndrome: amantadine, bromocriptine (Parlodel), dantrolene (Dantrium).

Antimanic and Mood-Stabilizing Agents Minimize Extreme Shifts in Emotions Between Mania and Depression.

Mechanism of Action	Examples	Nontherapeutic Effects
Lithium Affects neurotransmitters dopamine, serotonin, norepinephrine, acetylcholine, and GABA.	lithium carbonate	• Headache, fatigue, recent memory loss, anorexia, N&V, diarrhea, muscle weakness, ↑ BP, dizziness. • Teratogenic effect during first trimester. • *Toxicity:* Slurred speech, ataxia, tremors, disorientation, confusion, severe thirst, cogwheel rigidity, dilute urine, tinnitus, respiratory depression, and coma.
CNS agents, antiseizure agents Action varies depending on med.	carbamazepine (Tegretol) gabapentin (Neurontin) lamotrigine (Lamictal) topiramate (Topamax) valproates (Depakene) Depakote, Depacon)	• Drowsiness, fatigue, headache, nausea, blurred vision, psychomotor slowing. • May cause ↑ WBCs and ↑ platelets.

Nursing Care

- **Lithium**
  - Teach effect may take 1–2 weeks, take with meals to ↑ GI irritation, not to crush or chew medication.
  - Maintain fluid and Na intake because dehydration and hyponatremia may cause toxicity.
  - Assess therapeutic blood levels (0.15–1.5 mEq/L) weekly and then every 2–3 months; has narrow therapeutic window.

- **CNS and antiseizure agents:**
  - Teach tablets and sustained-release tablets are swallowed whole, chewable tablets are chewed, and carbonated beverages are not used to dilute elixir.
  - Avoid hazardous activities; protect from injury.
  - Monitor CBC and platelet counts routinely.

Medications for Attention Deficit Hyperactivity: Decrease Hyperactivity and Distractibility; Increase Alertness and Ability to Focus

Mechanism of Action	Examples	Nontherapeutic Effects
CNS stimulants Stimulate areas of CNS, mainly cerebral cortex.	methylphenidate (Concerta, Ritalin)	• Anorexia, insomnia, hypersensitivity, tachycardia, palpitations, HTN, restlessness, weight loss, growth suppression. • May cause paradoxical hyperactivity.
Nonstimulant norepinephrine reuptake inhibitor Inhibits norepinephrine uptake and transport	atomoxetine (Strattera)	Headache, insomnia, anorexia, vomiting, abdominal pain, cough, irritability, aggression, impotence.

Nursing Care
- Give 30–45 min before meals to ↑ food intake before anorexia occurs.
- Give 6 hr before sleep to ↓ sleep disturbances.
- Obtain baseline and periodic weight for ↑ or ↓ because dose is based on weight.
- Assess for S&S of depression or aggression; may require stopping medication.
- Inform school nurse and teacher of medication regimen.
- Teach that a drug holiday may be prescribed to assess progress and ↓ dependence.
- Withdraw gradually with medical supervision.
- *CNS stimulants:*
  - Teach duration is 3–6 hr; 8 hr for sustained-release forms.
  - Teach to not chew or crush sustained-release tablets.
- Strattera:
  - Teach duration is 12–24 hr.

Nontherapeutic Effects of Psychotropic Medications

Agranulocytosis
- S&S of infection: Fever, sore throat, cough.
- Urinary frequency, urgency due to UTI.

Anticholinergic Effects
- Dry mouth, urinary retention, constipation, blurred vision, ↑ P.

Cardiac Toxicity
- S&S of heart failure: ↓ BP, dysrhythmias, SOB, fatigue, ↑ weight, edema.

CNS Depression
- Drowsiness, sedation, orthostatic hypotension.

Peripheral CNS Stimulation (Sympathomimetic)
- ↑ P, ↑ BP, tremor, dysrhythmias.
- Restlessness, nightmares, insomnia, confusion.

Extrapyramidal Side Effects (EPS)
- *Akathisia:* Motor agitation, inability to rest or relax, pacing, restless legs, compulsive movements.
- *Dystonia:* Severe muscle spasms of back, neck, face, tongue.
- *Parkinsonism:* Tremor, muscle rigidity, bradykinesia, masklike facies, stooped posture, shuffling gait **(cogwheel gait),** drooling, restlessness.
- *Tardive dyskinesia:* Involuntary movements of tongue and face such as rolling or protrusion of tongue, lip smacking, teeth grinding, chewing motions, tics; movements disappear during sleep.

Hepatotoxicity
- Altered liver function studies, jaundice.

Hypersensitivity
- Rash, fever, arthralgia, urticaria.

Hypertensive Crisis
- Caused by high-dose antipsychotic medications or drug interactions.
- Headache, palpitations, stiff neck, photophobia, nausea, flushing, diaphoresis, dysrhythmias, death.

Hyponatremia
- N&V, diarrhea, fasciculations, stupor, seizures.

Neuroleptic Malignant Syndrome
- Caused by dopamine blockade in hypothalamus due to ↑ or prolonged dose of antipsychotic medications.

- ↑ temp (cardinal sign), diaphoresis, muscle rigidity, drowsiness, unstable BP, ↓ ventilation, dysrhythmias.

Serotonin Syndrome
- Caused by high dose of antidepressants; can be fatal.
- Confusion, anxiety, hyperpyrexia, ataxia, restlessness, tremors, hypertension, sweating.

Sexual Dysfunction
- ↓ libido, ↓ ability to reach orgasm, delayed ejaculation, impotence, cessation of menses or ovulation.

Herb-Drug Interactions

Herb/Use	Interactions
Echinacea Anti-infective, antipyretic.	↑ hepatotoxicity with amiodarone, anabolic steroids, ketoconazole, and methotrexate.
Feverfew Migraine headache.	↑ bleeding potential with aspirin, heparin, NSAIDs, and warfarin (Coumadin).
Garlic Lipid-lowering agent.	↑ bleeding potential with aspirin, NSAIDs, and warfarin. ↑ hypoglycemic effect of insulin and oral hypoglycemics.
Ginger Antiemetic.	↑ bleeding potential with aspirin, heparin, NSAIDs and warfarin.
Ginkgo Antiplatelet agent, CNS stimulant.	↑ bleeding potential with aspirin, heparin, NSAIDs and warfarin. ↓ effect of anticonvulsants, tricyclic antidepressants.
Ginseng ↑ stamina, ↑ immune response, ↑ appetite, antidepressant.	↓ anticoagulant effect of warfarin, ↑ hypoglycemic effect of insulin and oral hypoglycemics. ↑ digoxin toxicity, ↓ effect of diuretics, ↑ effect of CNS depressants.
Kava kava Antianxiety agent, sedative, hypnotic.	↑ sedation with barbiturates, CNS depressants, and benzodiazepines. ↑ dystonia with phenothiazines.

Continued

Herb/Use	Interactions
St. John's wort. Antidepressant.	• ↓ sedation with CNS depressants. • ↑ effect of cyclosporine, reserpine, and theophylline. • ↑ anticoagulant effect of warfarin and dabigatran (Pradaxa). • ↓ antiretroviral effect of protease inhibitors. • May cause serotonin syndrome with tricyclics and SSRIs. • May cause hypertensive crisis with MAO inhibitors.
Valerian. Antianxiety agent, sedative, hypnotic.	• ↓ sedation with barbiturates, benzodiazepines, and CNS depressants.

Medication Administration

Medication Administration: Key Points

Five Rights of Medication Administration	Patient Rights
• **Right patient** (check armband; date of birth; follow agency policy). • **Right medication.** • **Right dose.** • **Right route.** • **Right time.**	• Right to refuse medication. • Right to be educated. • Right to administration by knowledgeable, licensed person. • Right to be assessed before administration and evaluated after administration. • Right to have appropriate documentation.

Triple-Check Before Administration

■ *First:* Check label when removing from storage.
■ *Second:* Compare medication label to medication administration record (MAR).
■ *Third:* Check again after medication preparation, before administration.

Patient Teaching
- Assess patient attitude and ability for self-administration.
- Provide clear oral and written instructions; use understandable language.
- Include family members when appropriate.
- Evaluate learning; obtain return demonstration.
- Teach significant information:
  - Generic and trade name, purpose, therapeutic effect.
  - Dose, route, frequency, and when to take as-needed (prn) medications.
  - Nontherapeutic effects and what to do if S&S occur.
  - How to store medications, to take with or without food; pre- and postadministration assessments; and what to do if a dose is missed.

Safe Medication Administration

Preadministration Activities
- Check clinical record for known allergies.
- Obtain history of prescription and OTC medications.
- Confirm written order; repeat back and have a witness for verbal or phone orders.
- Be informed; check sources when unfamiliar with medication.
- Investigate compatibilities and interactions.
- Question overdose, subtherapeutic dose, medication duplication, extended use, medication order without indication.

Administration Activities
- Verify order against MAR.
- Calculate medication dosage; have another nurse double-check calculation.
- Follow rights of medication administration and triple-check procedure.
- Do not rush patient; ensure oral medications are ingested.
- Record medications given; document reasons for nonadministered medications.
- Identify therapeutic and nontherapeutic responses.
- Notify primary health-care provider of concerns or if patient vomits within 10 min of ingestion.

Safety and Legal Issues
- Do not borrow medications from another patient.
- Give only medications personally prepared.
- Do not leave medications at bedside.
- Double-lock controlled medications; have wasted controlled medications witnessed.
- Use filtered needle when drawing medications from an ampule.

- Crush medications and mix with smallest amount of applesauce to facilitate ingestion of entire dose; do not crush enteric or time-release medications.
- Document after, not before, medication is given; document and report medication errors.

Factors Affecting Medication Therapy

- **Development level:**
  - *Infants:* Immaturity of liver and kidneys require ↓ dose.
  - *Older adults:* ↓ liver and kidney function → accumulation; ↓ circulation and gastric function → ↓ medication absorption; ↑ medications (polypharmacy) ↑ interactions.
  - *Pregnancy:* May cause abnormal fetal development **(teratogenic).**
- **Diet:** Nutrients can ↑ or ↓ absorption or action of medication.
- **Gender:** Distribution of body fat, fluid, and hormones may affect medication action.
- **Environment:** Cold temperature can ↑ peripheral vasoconstriction; warm temperature can ↑ vasodilation; noise can ↑ effect of sedatives and analgesics.
- **Pathology:** ↓ liver or kidney function can cause ↑ medication accumulation; ↑ gastric or circulatory function can cause ↓ medication absorption.
- **Time of administration:** ↑ absorption on empty stomach; given with food to ↓ GI distress; circadian and sleep cycles can affect response.
- **Body weight:** Dose calculated by patient's weight or body surface area.
- **Genetic/ethnic/culture:** Usual dose may be toxic; herbal agents may ↑ or ↓ medication action; Asians may need ↓ dose of antipsychotic and antianxiety medications due to slower metabolism of these medications; black patients may need ↑ dose of antihypertensives.
- **Psychological:** Patient's positive or negative expectations can ↑ or ↓ response.

Effects of Medications

- **Adverse effect:** Severe side effect or toxicity.
- **Allergic reaction:** Immunological reaction.
- **Anaphylactic reaction:** Hypersensitive, life-threatening reaction.
- **Cumulative effect:** Excessive level of medication in body when intake is higher than metabolism or excretion.
- **Drug abuse:** Inappropriate intake of a medication.
- **Drug dependence:** Psychological or physiological need to take a medication.

- **Drug habituation:** Mild form of psychological dependence.
- **Drug interaction:** When one medication alters the effect of one or more medications.
- **Drug tolerance:** Requiring ↑ dose to achieve therapeutic effect.
- **Drug toxicity:** Dangerous effect due to excessive dose.
- **Idiosyncratic effect:** Unexpected or unique response.
- **Inhibiting effect:** One medication decreases effect of another medication.
- **Potentiating:** One medication adds to, prolongs, or ↑ action of another medication.
- **Side effect:** Predictable nontherapeutic effect that is tolerable.
- **Synergistic effect:** Combined effect of two medications is greater than when effect of each are added together.
- **Therapeutic effect:** Reason medication is prescribed; desired effect.

Medication Administration Routes

Route	Advantages (Pro) and Disadvantages (Con)	Nursing Care
Buccal Tablet or troche held between cheek and gum until dissolved. Local or systemic effect, depending on med. Absorbed within min.	**Pro:** Rapid relief. **Con:** Remains until dissolved; can be swallowed, chewed, or aspirated accidentally.	• Alternate cheeks to avoid mucosal irritation. • Warn not to chew or swallow tablet or sleep until dissolved to ↓ risk of aspiration.
Nasogastric tube (NGT), gastrostomy tube (GT, PEG) Instillation of med via a tube into stomach.	**Pro:** Used for ↓ gag reflex and unconscious patients. **Con:** Risk for aspiration; requires enteral tube and special equipment.	• Elevate head of bed (HOB); ensure placement of tube in stomach by aspirating gastric contents; clear tube with 30 mL of water; insert med through tube; clear tube with 30 mL of water after. • Assess for aspiration.

Continued

Route	Advantages (Pro) and Disadvantages (Con)	Nursing Care
Inhalation medications Dispersed through aerosolized solution or powder that penetrates airways, rapidly promoting absorption. MDI: metered-dose inhaler. NPA: nonpressurized aerosol nebulizer. DPI: dry powdered inhaler.	**Pro**: Rapid effect; can be given to unconscious patient. Use of spacer/extender with MDI ↓ particle size, promoting ↑ absorption and less droplets on tongue. **Con**: Can cause undesired systemic effects. Equipment needs to be cleaned and stored. Patient with ↓ cognition, infants, or children may be unable to follow directions. MDI: Requires coordination with inhalation and device compression.	**MDI** • Shake canister before each depression. • Exhale through pursed lips. • Hold 2 cm from mouth or insert mouthpiece beyond teeth with lips around mouthpiece (may use spacer). • Depress device while inhaling slowly and deeply; hold breath 5–10 sec. • Exhale slowly via pursed lips; wait 1–2 min between inhalations. • Rinse mouth and clean MDI afterward. **NPA** • Insert dose in chamber. • Breathe in and out with lips closed around mouthpiece. • Take deep breath every 5 breaths. • Repeat until no misting. Rinse mouth and clean equipment afterward. **DPI** • Prepare inhaler for use. • Close mouth around mouthpiece. • Take deep breath; dose in chamber is aerosolized when inhaled. • Hold breath 5–15 sec. Rinse mouth and clean DPI afterward.

Route	Advantages (Pro) and Disadvantages (Con)	Nursing Care
Intradermal (ID) Solution injected into dermis just under epidermis. Slow absorption. Volume 0.1–0.3 mL.	**Pro:** Used for allergy testing. **Con:** Pierces skin.	• Use standard precautions. • Assess for allergic or anaphylactic reaction when used for allergy testing.
Intramuscular (IM) Solution injected into muscle. Onset 3–5 min. Volume 1–3 mL.	**Pro:** Used when oral route is contraindicated; more rapidly absorbed than oral, topical, or sub-Q. **Con:** Pierces skin; more tissue damage than sub-Q. Requires adequate peripheral circulation. Can cause anxiety.	• Use standard precautions. • Use sterile technique. • Position patient to access injection site. • Landmark sites. • Rotate sites.
Intravenous (IV) solution Injected into intravascular compartment via a vein. Immediate onset.	**Pro:** Immediate therapeutic effect. **Con:** More costly than oral; can cause anxiety.	• Use standard precautions. • Use sterile technique. • Administer IV push, intermittent, continuous titrated drips as prescribed. • Change tubing every 24–72 hr and site 3–7 days as per agency policy.
Oral (PO) Taken by mouth in tablet, capsule, or liquid form. Absorbed in GI tract. Onset 30–45 min.	**Pro:** Convenient, does not invade skin, economical; less psychological stress than other routes. **Con:** May irritate gastric mucosa, have bad taste or odor, discolor or erode teeth, cause aspiration.	• Elevate HOB to ensure safe swallowing. • Pace intake to ↓ aspiration. • Crush meds and mix with food if patient has dysphagia; do not crush extended-release and enteric-coated meds; obtain liquid form if available.

Continued

Route	Advantages (Pro) and Disadvantages (Con)	Nursing Care
	Contraindications: Vomiting, dysphasia, unconsciousness, continuous NG suction.	Obtain prescription for alternate route.
Rectal (PR) Suppository or solution inserted into anus. Slow absorption; local or systemic effect.	**Pro:** Used if oral route is contraindicated. **Con:** Patient embarrassment; absorption unpredictable. **Contraindications:** Rectal surgery or rectal bleeding.	• Use standard precautions. • Position patient in lateral or Sims position for insertion.
Subcutaneous (Sub-Q) Solution inserted into tissue just below skin. Onset 3–20 min. Volume ≤1 mL.	**Pro:** Faster than oral. **Con:** Pierces skin; can be irritating to tissue.	• Use standard precautions. • Use sterile technique. • Landmark sites. • Rotate injection sites.
Sublingual (SL) Under tongue. Rapid absorption.	**Pro:** Immediate therapeutic response. **Con:** Can be swallowed, chewed, or aspirated accidentally.	• Instruct to keep liquid or tablet under tongue. • Warn not to chew or swallow tablet or sleep until it is absorbed.
Swish and Spit Solution dispersed throughout oral cavity and expelled from mouth. **Swish and Swallow** Solution dispersed throughout oral cavity and swallowed.	**Pro:** Easy and inexpensive to implement; provides local effect. **Con:** Some patients may not be able to follow directions to swish solution; may swallow the solution meant for a swish and spit; may be accidentally aspirated.	• Instruct to keep lips closed and by puffing cheeks in and out move solution around entire oral cavity and then: • *Swish and spit:* Expel solution from mouth. • *Swish and swallow:* Swallow solution.

Route	Advantages (Pro) and Disadvantages (Con)	Nursing Care
Transdermal Via the skin (percutaneous). Prolonged absorption.	**Pro:** Prolonged systemic effect; limited side effects; avoids GI irritation. **Con:** Residue may irritate skin or soil clothes.	• Wear gloves to ↓ self-contamination. • Use site indicated by manufacturer such as chest, upper arms, anterior thighs. • Rotate sites. • Avoid impaired skin; use hairless area to ensure patch contact. • Wash site after removing patch.
Vaginal Inserted into vaginal vault.	**Pro:** Local effect. **Con:** Limited use; patient embarrassment.	• Use standard precautions. • Clean perineum before and after insertion. • Position in dorsal recumbent or Sims position. • Lubricate applicator or finger with water-soluble gel. • Insert applicator into vagina to depth recommended by manufacturer and depress plunger; insert suppository full length of index finger. • Instruct to remain supine for 15 min. • Wash and dry applicator.

Intramuscular Injection Sites and Z-Track Method for Giving IM Injections

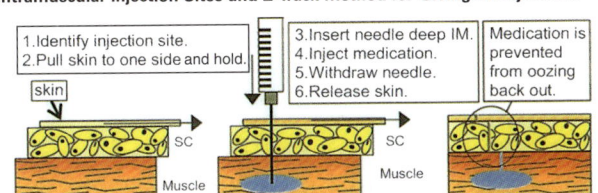

1. Identify injection site.
2. Pull skin to one side and hold.

skin

3. Insert needle deep IM.
4. Inject medication.
5. Withdraw needle.
6. Release skin.

Medication is prevented from oozing back out.

SC

Muscle

SC

Muscle

	ID	Sub-Q	IM
Site	Inner forearm, chest, and back.	Outer upper arm, anterior thigh, abdomen.	Gluteus, vastus lateralis, deltoid muscles.
Gauge	27–30	25–28	23
Length	1/4–3/8 inch	5/8 inch	1–1½ inch
Angle	10–15°	90° 45° for very thin patients.	90°
Volume	0.1–0.2 mL	0.5–1 mL	Up to 3 mL; small muscles (deltoid) no more than 1 mL.

Sub-Q Heparin and Low Molecular Weight Anticoagulant Injections

Site	Gauge and Angle	Aspirate	Massage Site
Abdomen, posterior upper arm, low back, thigh, and upper back.	25–26 gauge, 3/8 inch. 90° angle (45° if patient is underweight).	No	No

Injection Techniques

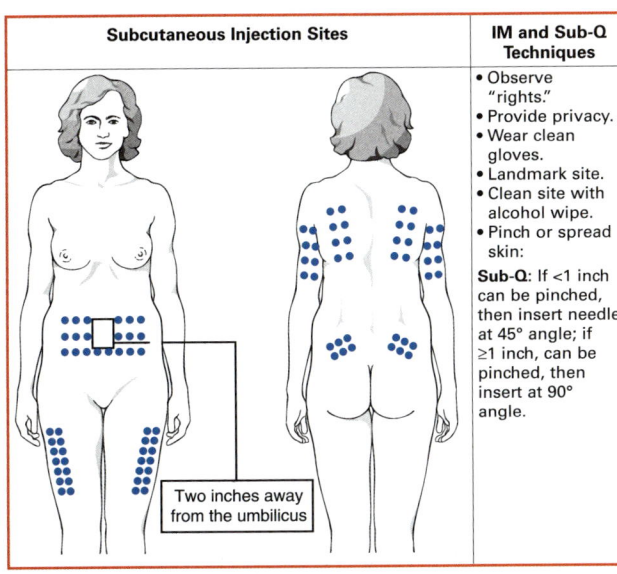

Subcutaneous Injection Sites	IM and Sub-Q Techniques

IM and Sub-Q Techniques
- Observe "rights."
- Provide privacy.
- Wear clean gloves.
- Landmark site.
- Clean site with alcohol wipe.
- Pinch or spread skin:

Sub-Q: If <1 inch can be pinched, then insert needle at 45° angle; if ≥1 inch, can be pinched, then insert at 90° angle.

Two inches away from the umbilicus

IM Injection Sites	Injection Techniques

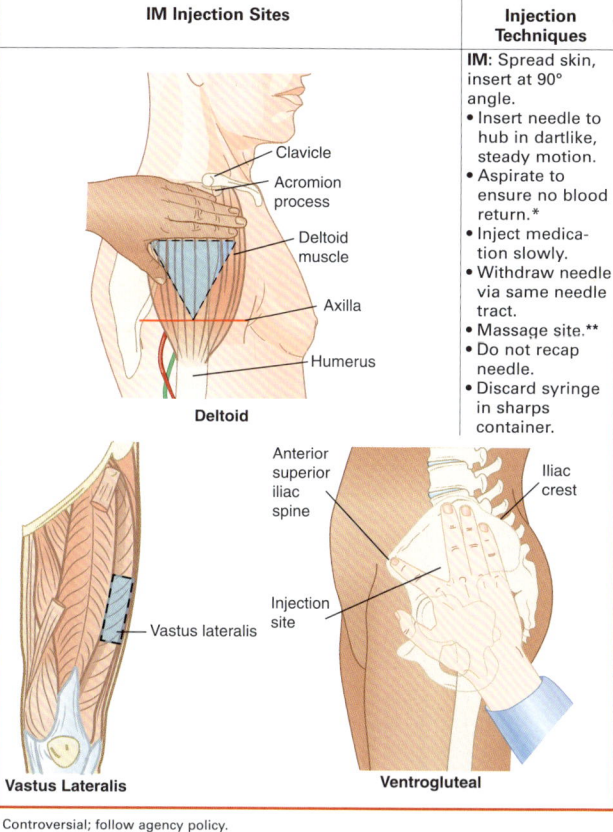

IM: Spread skin, insert at 90° angle.
- Insert needle to hub in dartlike, steady motion.
- Aspirate to ensure no blood return.*
- Inject medication slowly.
- Withdraw needle via same needle tract.
- Massage site.**
- Do not recap needle.
- Discard syringe in sharps container.

Clavicle
Acromion process
Deltoid muscle
Axilla
Humerus

Deltoid

Anterior superior iliac spine
Iliac crest
Injection site

Vastus Lateralis

Vastus lateralis

Ventrogluteal

* Controversial; follow agency policy.
** Do not massage when injecting heparin or insulin, or when using Z-tract technique.

- Assess integrity of primary IV site such as no S&S of infiltration or inflammation; ensure primary set is patent and not expired.
- Ensure compatibility of primary solution and med in IVPB.
- Attach secondary tubing to IVPB bag; flush tubing without wasting any solution; clamp tubing.
- Hang IVPB bag higher than primary IV bag; primary IV bag may need a hook to extend bag lower.
- Connect secondary tubing to primary set using port most distal from patient.
- Open IVPB tubing clamp, set rate via primary set roller clamp.

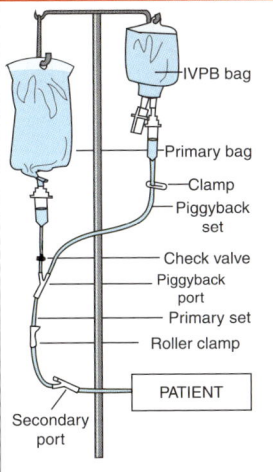

IVPB bag

Primary bag

Clamp

Piggyback set

Check valve

Piggyback port

Primary set

Roller clamp

PATIENT

Secondary port

Complication	Nursing Assessment	Nursing Care
Infiltration IV fluid escapes into subcutaneous tissue; ↓ or no fluids infusing.	Assess site for swelling, pale, cool to touch No blood return when IV bag is held lower than insertion site.	• Discontinue IV; apply ordered warm compress; restart in new site. • *Prevention:* Discourage movement of limb with IV.

Continued

Complication	Nursing Assessment	Nursing Care
Phlebitis Inflammation of vein. **Thrombus** Blood clot; IV flow may stop due to obstruction.	Assess for red line or burning pain along course of vein, heat, and swelling.	• Discontinue IV; apply ordered warm compress; do not massage or rub affected area; restart in new site; notify primary health-care provider. • *Prevention:* Discourage movement of limb with IV; flush as per policy; change and rotate sites as per policy (generally every 72 hr).
Fluid overload Patient cannot tolerate rate of infusion; rate is faster than ordered.	Assess for hypervolemia: Bounding; ↑ P; ↑ BP; ↑ R; lung base crackles; dyspnea; distended neck veins.	• ↓ IV rate and notify primary health-care provider. • If experiencing respiratory complications: ↑ HOB; provide oxygen at 2 L/min. • *Prevention:* Assess response first 15 min frequently after hanging new solution; assess rate regularly; use time tape and volume control device.
Incorrect solution Solution other than what was ordered is infusing.	Check IV order with hanging IV fluid.	• ↓ IV rate to maintain patency; immediately hang correct solution; notify primary health-care provider; complete incident report. • *Prevention:* Verify solution with order 3 times before hanging IV solution.

Complication	Nursing Assessment	Nursing Care
IV rate is too slow Volume absorbed is ↓ than volume ordered.	Inspect factors affecting flow such as kinks, lying on tubing, dependent loops; IV bag too low; arm position that impairs flow rate.	• Change IV site if infiltrated; remove tubing from under patient; coil tubing on bed; reposition arm; maintain at ordered rate (do not increase rate because it may precipitate fluid overload). • *Prevention:* Assess flow rate routinely, use time tape, position bag 3 feet above IV site, coil tubing on bed surface, discourage movement of limb with IV.
Air embolus Air in intravascular compartment.	Assess for respiratory distress, ↑ P, cyanosis, ↓ BP, ↓ LOC.	• Secure system to prevent entry of air; place patient on left side in modified Trendelenburg position; continue to assess VS, O_2 sat. • Notify primary health-care provider. • *Prevention:* Flush IV lines of air before use; assess integrity of system frequently.
Sepsis Systemic infection.	Assess for ↑ VS and/or red, tender, insertion site.	• Follow agency guidelines for specimen collection for cultures such as blood or exudate. • Notify primary health-care provider. • *Prevention:* Use meticulous sterile technique.

Medication Calculation Formulas

IV Drop Rate Formula

- Drop factor equals number of drops per mL delivered by IV tubing.

$$\text{Drops per minute} = \frac{\text{total mL}}{\text{total time in minutes}} \times \text{drop factor}$$
$$\frac{\text{(total volume in drops)}}{\frac{60 \text{ minutes}}{1 \text{ hour}} \times X}$$

Conversion of Pounds to Kilograms (kg)

- Solve for X by cross multiplying.
- Divide both sides of resulting equation by the number in front of the X.
- Reduce to lowest terms to achieve child's weight in kg.

$$\text{child's weight in pounds} = x \text{ kg} \quad \frac{2.2 \text{ pounds}}{1 \text{ kg}}$$

Ratio and Proportion Formulas

- Ordered dose and dose on hand must be in same unit of measure.
- **Formulas 1 and 2:** Solve for X by cross multiplying.
- **Formula 3:** Solve for X by multiplying the means and the extremes.
- Divide both sides of all resulting equations by the number in front of the X.
- Reduce to lowest terms to achieve the quantity of dose.

$$\#1 \quad \frac{\text{desired}}{\text{have}} = \frac{\text{ordered dose}}{\text{dose on hand}} = \frac{X \text{ quantity desired}}{\text{quantity on hand}}$$

$$\#2 \quad \frac{\text{quantity on hand}}{\text{dose on hand}} = \frac{X \text{ quantity desired}}{\text{ordered dose}}$$

$$\#3 \quad \text{dose on hand} : \text{quantity on hand} :: \text{ordered dose} : X \text{ quantity desired}$$
$$\text{(extreme)} \qquad \text{(means)} \qquad \text{(means)} \qquad \text{(extreme)}$$

Pediatric Dosage Calculations

Body Surface Area (BSA) Method

■ Estimate the child's BSA in square meters (m²) by using a BSA chart (nomogram).*

■ The BSA chart consists of three columns. The left column is height, the middle column is body surface area, and the right column is weight. These numbers increase from the bottom to the top of each column.

■ Draw a straight line from the child's height in the left column to the child's weight in the right column. The number found where the line crosses the middle column is the child's estimated BSA.

■ The BSA should be used in the formula for the body surface area method to calculate a pediatric dose.

$$\text{Pediatric dose in mg} = \frac{\text{Child's BSA in square meters (m}^2) \times \text{Adult dose in mg}}{1.73 \text{ m}^2}$$

Young's Rule: Age-Based (1–12 years) Method

$$\text{child's dose} = \frac{\text{child's age (in years)}}{\text{child's age (in years + 12)}} \quad X \quad \text{average adult dose}$$

*Deglin, Vallerand, Sanoski; *Davis's Drug Guide for Nurses*, 12th Ed., 2011; F.A. Davis, Co., Philadelphia; Appendix F, Body Surface Area Nomograms, p.1409.

Test Analysis Tools

■ This tab includes tips and analysis tools that will help you pass the NCLEX-RN. Seven tools are included to help you analyze your test performance:
1. Performance Trends
2. Information Processing Errors
3. Knowledge Deficits: Universal Information
4. Knowledge Deficits: Medical-Surgical Nursing
5. Knowledge Deficits: Pediatric Nursing
6. Knowledge Deficits: Childbearing Nursing
7. Knowledge Deficits: Mental Health and Psychiatric Nursing

■ Performance trends and information-processing errors focus on the process of test-taking, and corrective-action plans are presented to address your identified deficits.

■ Knowledge deficits: Universal information focuses on content common to all disciplines in nursing practice.

■ Four tools concerning knowledge deficits (medical-surgical, pediatric, childbearing, and mental health/psychiatric nursing) focus on discipline-specific content.

Instructions for Information-Processing Errors and Knowledge-Deficit Tools

■ First look over each tool. After taking and scoring your test, use the tools to help you identify your area of weakness.

■ Complete all tools in the same way:
1. Place the number of a question you got wrong in a box in the top row under **question number**.
2. Identify the **processing error** or **knowledge category** associated with your error in the left column.
3. Put a mark in the box where the row and column intersect on the chart; follow the first three steps for all your wrong answers.

4. Tally the total number of marks for each row in the last column on the right; after you identify clusters of deficits, see the tool **Corrective Action Plan** and follow the suggestions addressing your specific deficit.

Instructions for Performance Trends

■ Answer the following questions to identify opportunities to improve your test-taking skills:

Performance Trends

• I am able to focus with little distraction.	Yes ( ) No ( )
• I feel calm and in control.	Yes ( ) No ( )
• I effectively use test-taking techniques to reduce options.	Yes ( ) No ( )
• I change answers from wrong to right.	Yes ( ) No ( )
• I have no error clusters: beginning, middle, or end of exam.	Yes ( ) No ( )

■ If you answered **No** to any of these questions, see the tool **Corrective Action Plan**.

Information-Processing Errors

Knowledge Category	Question Numbers								
Stem									
• Missed negative polarity									
• Missed word setting priority									
• Missed important clues									
• Misinterpreted information									
• Missed central point, theme									
• Read into the question									
• Missed step in nursing process									
• Incompletely analyzed stem									

Continued

Information-Processing Errors—cont'd

Knowledge Category	Question Numbers									
Stem										
• Did not understand question										
• Did not know the content										
Options										
• Selected the answer too quickly										
• Misidentified the priority										
• Misinterpreted information										
• Read into options										
• Did not know the content										
• Misapplied concepts, principles										
• Transcribed incorrectly										

Knowledge Deficits: Universal Information

Knowledge Category	Question Numbers									
• A&P and pathophysiology										
• Basic care (including pain)										
• Community care										
• Complementary, alternative care										
• Death/dying/loss/grief										
• Emergency care										
• Fluid and electrolyte balance										
• Growth and development										
• Inflammation/infection										
• Leadership and management										
• Legal and ethical issues										

Knowledge Deficits: Universal Information—cont'd

Knowledge Category	Question Numbers							
• Perioperative								
• Pharmacology								
• Psychosociocultural and communication								
• Safety (physical/ microbiological)								
• Teaching and learning								
Nursing Process								
• Assessment								
• Analysis and diagnosis								
• Planning								
• Implementation								
• Evaluation								

Knowledge Deficits: Medical-Surgical Nursing

Knowledge Category	Question Numbers							
• Cardiac								
• Endocrine								
• GI, accessory organs of digestion (gallbladder, liver, pancreas)								
• GI, upper (mouth, esophagus, stomach)								
• GI, lower (small and large intestines)								
• Hematological, immunological, lymphatic								
• Integumentary								

Continued

Knowledge Deficits: Medical-Surgical Nursing—cont'd

Knowledge Category	Question Numbers							
• Musculoskeletal								
• Neoplastic								
• Neurological								
• Peripheral vascular								
• Reproductive (female)								
• Reproductive (male)								
• Respiratory								
• Urinary								
• Other								

Knowledge Deficits: Pediatric Nursing

Knowledge Category	Question Numbers							
• Cardiac disease (congenital, acquired)								
• Endocrine								
• GI, accessory organs of digestion (gallbladder, liver, pancreas)								
• GI, upper (mouth, esophagus, stomach)								
• GI, lower (small, large intestines)								
• Genitourinary								
• Growth and development								
• Health promotion and immunization								
• Hematological, immunological, lymphatic								

Knowledge Deficits: Pediatric Nursing—cont'd

Knowledge Category	Question Numbers								
• Integumentary									
• Musculoskeletal									
• Neoplastic									
• Neurological									
• Peripheral vascular									
• Respiratory									
• Other									

Knowledge Deficits: Childbearing Nursing

Knowledge Category	Question Numbers								
• Family (adjustment/loss)									
• Diagnostic testing									
• Nutrition: Maternal, infant (breast/formula)									
• Prenatal care									
• Intrapartal care (labor/birth)									
• High-risk pregnancy									
• Obstetric emergencies									
• Postpartum care									
• Healthy newborn									
• High-risk newborn									
• Other									

Knowledge Deficits: Mental Health and Psychiatric Nursing

Knowledge Category	Question Numbers							
• Crisis/stress management								
• Defense mechanisms								
• Dysfunctional behavior patterns								
• Therapeutic communication								
• Treatment modalities								
• Violence (sexual/domestic/ suicide)								
• Other								
Disorders								
• Anxiety disorders								
• Attention deficit and disruptive behavior								
• Cognitive disorders (dementia/ delirium)								
• Dissociative disorders								
• Eating disorders								
• Factitious disorders								
• Grief and loss								
• Mood disorders (depressive/ bipolar)								
• Personality disorders								
• Pervasive developmental disorders								
• Schizophrenia								
• Sexual and gender identity disorders								
• Somatoform disorders								
• Substance abuse disorders								

Corrective Action Plan

Performance Trends

■ Implement recommendations if you scored **No** on the Performance Trends tool.
  1. Be comfortable, rested, sit in area free of distractions; wear earplugs.
  2. Develop a positive mental attitude (challenge negative thoughts, use positive self-talk: "I can do this!").
     ■ Regain control (use deep breathing, imagery, muscle relaxation).
     ■ Desensitize yourself to fear response (practice test-taking).
     ■ Establish control on day of exam (manage routine, travel, environment, supplies).
     ■ Stop exam, take a break, and regain control; do not get bogged down on answering questions on content you do not know—move on; overprepare for the exam.
  3. Practice test-taking tips presented in TIPS Tab.
  4. If you change more answers from right to wrong on practice tests, **do not** change your first answer unless you are absolutely certain that the new answer is correct.
  5. Use anxiety-reducing techniques during the exam at times when error clusters appeared in practice; if due to fatigue, stop exam and take a short break; work at practice tests longer to increase stamina.

Information-Processing Errors

■ Practice test-taking tips presented in TIPS Tab.
■ For more detail see Nugent, *Test Success: Test-Taking Techniques for Beginning Nursing Students,* F. A. Davis, Philadelphia.

Knowledge Deficits: All Areas

■ Focus study on clustered gaps in knowledge.
■ Review notes, text, computer-assisted instruction, videos, and practice test questions with rationales; use study workbooks and computer programs.
■ Do not waste time studying areas you know.
■ Explore the F. A. Davis Notes series for a title that reviews the topic in more depth than is presented in NCLEX-RN Notes (e.g., Psych, MedSurg, Lab, MED, Ortho, Nutri, ECG, IV Therapy, RN).

Illustration Credits

Tab 2: Wong-Baker FACES Pain Rating Scale. From Wong D. L., Hockenberry-Eaton M., Willson D., Winkelstein M. L., Schwartz P. *Wong's Essentials of Pediatric Nursing*, 6th ed. Mosby, St. Louis, MO, 2001, p. 1301. Copyrighted by Mosby. Reprinted by permission.

Tab 4: The Centers for Disease Control.

Tab 7: Wilkinson J. M., and Treas L. S. *Fundamentals of Nursing Thinking, Doing and Caring*, vol. 2, 2nd ed. F. A. Davis, Philadelphia, 2011.

Davis's Notes
Your Handheld Clinical Companions

- Vital clinical information
- Portable and pocket-sized
- Easy-to-reference tabs

**NCLEX-RN® Content Review plus Q&A...
wherever you go!**

Here are the tips, strategies, techniques, and content you need to pass the NCLEX-RN® exam—all in one pocket-sized resource.

- Features tips to manage test-taking anxiety as well as specific strategies for answering multiple-choice and alternate-format questions.
- Codes all questions by client need, content area, cognitive domain, and difficulty level.
- Includes comprehensive rationales so you understand why your responses were correct or incorrect.
- Emphasizes critical thinking, study skills, and time management.
- Offers self-assessment test-analysis tools.
- Includes a Bonus Question Bank with 850 NCLEX-RN® questions.

Look for our other Davis's Notes and Pocket Guide titles
RNotes® • MedSurg Notes
NCLEX-RN® Alternate-Format Q&A

Visit us at www.FADavis.com

F.A. Davis Company • Independent Publishers Since 1879

ISBN 13: 978-0-8036-2913-4

9 780803 629134

Centimeters